Hearing Loss in Children: The Present and a Challenge for Future

Hearing Loss in Children: The Present and a Challenge for Future

Guest Editors

Gauri Mankekar
Lindsey Collins

MDPI

Basel • Beijing • Wuhan • Barcelona • Belgrade • Novi Sad • Cluj • Manchester

Guest Editors
Gauri Mankekar
Department of
Otolaryngology
Louisiana State Health
University Sciences Center
Shreveport, LA
USA

Lindsey Collins
Department of
Otolaryngology Head Neck
Surgery
LSU Health Shreveport
Shreveport, LA
USA

Editorial Office
MDPI AG
Grosspeteranlage 5
4052 Basel, Switzerland

This is a reprint of the Special Issue, published open access by the journal *Children* (ISSN 2227-9067), freely accessible at: https://www.mdpi.com/journal/children/special_issues/89S27115M7.

For citation purposes, cite each article independently as indicated on the article page online and as indicated below:

Lastname, A.A.; Lastname, B.B. Article Title. *Journal Name* **Year**, *Volume Number*, Page Range.

ISBN 978-3-7258-7342-5 (Hbk)
ISBN 978-3-7258-7343-2 (PDF)
https://doi.org/10.3390/books978-3-7258-7343-2

Contents

About the Editors

Gauri Mankekar

Gauri Mankekar, MD, PhD, FACS is a neurotologist at LSU Health, Ochsner LSU Health and the Overton Brooks VA Medical Center, Shreveport, Louisiana, USA. She provides comprehensive hearing healthcare for adult and pediatric patients. She completed her medical education at Seth GS Medical College and KEM Hospital, Mumbai, India, followed by a PhD from the University of Wuerzburg, Germany. She subsequently completed her Advanced Otology Fellowship at The Lady of the Lake, Baton Rouge, LA. Her focus is on the evaluation and surgical management of hearing loss, cochlear implantation, and implantable hearing devices.

Lindsey Collins

Lindsey Collins, AuD. CCC-A, is a clinical audiologist at Ochsner LSU Health in Shreveport, where she provides comprehensive hearing healthcare to adults and children. She earned her doctorate in audiology from Louisiana Tech University in 2023 and completed her clinical residency at Nemours Children's Hospital in Orlando, Florida. Dr. Collins specializes in diagnosing hearing loss across the lifespan and has experience evaluating patients for cochlear implant candidacy, as well as activating and programming their devices. She is skilled in fitting and programming a wide range of implantable technologies, including cochlear implants and bone-anchored hearing systems, and also provides care for hearing aid patients.

Preface

We are pleased to present this Special Issue on hearing loss in children. It aims to advance early detection and management, outlining causes, diagnostic challenges and emerging interventions in pediatric hearing loss, and is motivated by the need to improve outcomes for children with hearing loss. The Special Issue is addressed to clinicians, researchers and trainees.

Gauri Mankekar and Lindsey Collins
Guest Editors

children

MDPI

Article

Increasing Genetic Testing Uptake Through Workflow Optimization: A Quality Improvement Study in Pediatric Hearing Loss

Jennifer Coto [1,2], Julia Anne Morris [2,3], Valerie Yunis [2], Chrisanda Marie Sanchez [1,2], Xue Zhong Liu [1,2,*] and Ivette Cejas [1,2,*]

1 Department of Pediatrics, University of Miami, Miami, FL 33136, USA; jennifercoto@med.miami.edu (J.C.)
2 Department of Otolaryngology, University of Miami, Miami, FL 33136, USA
3 Morsani College of Medicine, University of South Florida, Tampa, FL 33620, USA
* Correspondence: x.liu1@med.miami.edu (X.Z.L.); icejas@med.miami.edu (I.C.)

Highlights

What are the main findings?

- Implementation of a standardized genetics referral protocol more than doubled documented referral rates for children with hearing loss in an otology and audiology clinic.
- Use of predefined referral pathways increased consistency in referral practices across providers and referral modalities.

What is the implication of the main finding?

- Structured referral pathways and brief provider education can meaningfully reduce gaps between guideline recommendations and real-world clinical practice.
- Quality improvement strategies offer a scalable approach to improving access to genetic evaluation and advancing precision care for pediatric hearing loss.

Abstract

Background/Objectives: Although genetic testing is recommended for pediatric hearing loss, referral rates within otology and audiology practices remain low. This study evaluated referral rates, referral pathways, and genetics appointment completion before and after implementation of a quality improvement (QI) referral protocol in an ethnically diverse pediatric cohort. Methods: Phase 1 (January–August 2023) included chart reviews of 88 pediatric patients with hearing loss to assess whether genetics referrals were made and completed. Data collected included demographics, referral modality (clinical note documentation, routed note to genetics, or direct referral order), and appointment status. In Phase 2 (September 2023–September 2024), a standardized referral protocol was implemented requiring all newly diagnosed patients to be referred using one of three predefined pathways. Providers received brief training and reminder cards. Chart reviews were then conducted for an additional 114 patients. Results: A total of 202 patients were included (Phase 1: $n = 88$; Phase 2: $n = 114$). Following protocol implementation, the proportion of patients with any documented genetics referral increased significantly (35.2% vs. 68.4%, $\chi^2 = 22.03$, $p < 0.001$). Referral order placement, documentation, and note routing increased across all referral modalities (all $p < 0.001$). Genetics appointment completion also improved significantly, from 11.4% in Phase 1 to 38.6% in Phase 2 ($p < 0.001$). Conclusions: Genetic referrals for pediatric hearing loss remain underutilized but improved substantially following implementation of a standardized referral protocol. These findings highlight the importance of optimizing referral pathways and providing ongoing provider education.

QI initiatives represent a practical strategy to enhance access to genetic evaluation and support precision care.

Keywords: hearing loss; pediatrics; genetic testing; quality improvement

1. Introduction

Hearing loss is the most common sensory disorder, affecting more than 430 million people worldwide, including 34 million children [1]. In developed countries, approximately 1.7 to 3 per 1000 children are born with detectable hearing loss, with prevalence increasing to approximately 3.5 per 1000 by adolescence [2,3]. In pediatric populations, 50–70% of hearing loss is attributable to genetic mutations [4,5]. These may be syndromic (~30%), where hearing loss occurs in combination with other systemic symptoms, such as in Usher, Pendred, Alport, or Jervell and Lange-Nielsen syndromes, or non-syndromic (~70%), with common variants including *GJB2*, *OTOF*, and *TMPRSS3* [5,6]. The burden on affected children and families is substantial. Hearing loss in children contributes to delays in speech and language development, reduced educational outcomes, and social isolation [5,7,8]. Furthermore, approximately 60% of educationally significant hearing loss is caused by genetic factors [6]. Therefore, the current study aimed to assess the impact of implementing a streamlined referral pathway within an otology and audiology practice on rates of genetic testing completion as part of a quality improvement (QI) initiative.

Importantly, children who receive early intervention with hearing amplification or cochlear implants (CI) have been shown to have improved long-term language outcomes [8–10]. Delayed diagnosis and intervention can worsen prognosis. Information regarding genetic diagnosis may further inform clinical decision-making by clarifying prognosis, supporting earlier determination of cochlear implant candidacy, and enabling intervention during critical periods of auditory and language neuroplasticity, which has been linked to improved CI outcomes [11], particularly in variants such as *GJB2* or *OTOF*, which are associated with better auditory performance post-implantation than other genetic causes [12].

Given the heterogeneity of hearing loss, involving more than 100 implicated genes and over 400 associated genetic syndromes, genetic testing has become essential to diagnostic evaluation [6]. The American College of Medical Genetics and Genomics (ACMG) recommends genetic testing for all children with hearing loss, citing benefits for clinical management, prognostic accuracy, genetic counseling, intervention planning, and targeted surveillance for syndromic comorbidities [6,13,14]. Other major organizations, including the Joint Committee on Infant Hearing (JCIH), the American Academy of Pediatrics (AAP), the American Speech-Language-Hearing Association (ASHA), and the International Pediatric Otolaryngology Group (IPOG), also endorse genetic testing for infants with hearing loss [14]. Beyond medical management, genetic testing provides critical counseling information by clarifying etiology, recurrence risk, and intervention options [4,5,15,16].

Genetic testing also enables early identification and monitoring of syndromic complications, such as progressive vision loss in Usher syndrome, kidney function in Alport syndrome, thyroid function in Pendred syndrome, or potentially life-threatening arrhythmias caused by QT prolongation in Jervell and Lange-Nielsen syndrome [5,13,16]. It is well established that genetic screening as early as possible is most effective in optimizing outcomes in these patients [5,15]. Advances in genetic testing technology, particularly the transition from Sanger sequencing to next-generation sequencing (NGS), have substantially improved access to comprehensive testing. NGS enables the simultaneous analysis of thousands of genes at a cost comparable to traditional single-gene approaches [16]. This expanded capacity is especially important for hearing loss, which is highly genetically heterogeneous, as broader panel-based testing increases diagnostic yield compared with targeted testing strategies [16,17].

Despite established professional guidelines and well-documented benefits of etiologic and genetic evaluation, genetic testing for pediatric hearing loss remains underutilized. Recent surveys indicate that fewer than half of providers routinely refer children with hearing loss for genetic testing, and many families are never offered testing at all [14,18]. Reported barriers include limited provider awareness, inconsistent referral practices, workflow inefficiencies, restricted access to genetic counseling, and insurance or cost-related concerns. Notably, these gaps persist even in well-resourced settings. At our large, multiethnic, university-based hospital system with an established multidisciplinary team that includes on-site genetics services, baseline referral rates remained suboptimal, suggesting that system-level workflow barriers—rather than resource availability alone—may impede appropriate testing.

To address this gap, we implemented a quality improvement (QI) initiative designed to standardize and streamline the genetics referral process within our otology and audiology practice. The primary aim was to increase the proportion of children with hearing loss referred for genetic evaluation by embedding a structured referral workflow into routine clinical care. To assess the impact of this intervention, we conducted a retrospective chart review comparing referral completion and testing outcomes before and after protocol implementation.

2. Materials and Methods

2.1. Procedures

As part of a QI initiative, a retrospective chart review was completed for patients seen at the Children's Hearing Program (CHP) at the University of Miami for patients under the age of 17 who had received a diagnosis of hearing loss from January 2023–August 2023 (Phase 1) and September 2023 to September 2024 (Phase 2). These two phases represented pre- and post-implementation periods for the quality improvement intervention. Phase 1 reflected usual care referral practices prior to protocol implementation, whereas Phase 2 captured outcomes after introduction of the standardized referral workflow, allowing comparison of referral rates before and after the intervention. Assignment to Phase 1 or Phase 2 was based solely on the date of the patient's diagnostic visit relative to the timing of protocol implementation. Hearing loss criteria included children with diagnosed unilateral or bilateral sensorineural (SNHL) mixed (MHL), or conductive (CHL) hearing loss. For the CHL inclusion, children were included if they were considered to have long-term or chronic CHL (e.g., microtia/atresia and other middle ear anomalies such as cholesteatoma or ossicular malformations). Children with transient otitis media were not referred for genetic evaluation. Exclusion criteria included patients who presented to clinic for reimplant or had explant surgeries and those who had undergone genetic testing elsewhere. Demographic variables extracted for each patient included demographic information (age, sex, ethnicity, race, language) along with medical information (insurance type, hearing loss degree, and device(s) used).

During Phase I, variables collected during the chart review included if a referral order for genetic testing was placed, if the chart was routed to the genetics team, and if any mention of a referral to genetics was made in the clinical note. For each of these variables, we also indicated which provider (i.e., otologist, audiologist, etc.) completed the task. Additionally, we extracted whether a genetics appointment was made, the status

https://doi.org/10.3390/children13020240

of the appointment (completed, no-show, or canceled), and whether a genetic mutation was identified.

After completion of Phase 1 data collection, a QI protocol was implemented to increase referral rates to genetics for patients newly diagnosed with hearing loss. The protocol introduced three standardized referral pathways that were applied to all patients at the time of diagnosis. Specifically, during the diagnostic appointment, providers were instructed to: (1) document the genetics referral in the recommendations section of the clinical note; (2) route the clinical note to the genetics team; and (3) place an electronic referral order for genetic testing.

To support implementation, audiologists and otologists received email communication outlining the updated referral procedures. The updated procedures were also discussed during a monthly department meeting and sufficient time was allocated for any questions by providers. In addition, laminated ID badge cards with simplified step-by-step instructions were distributed to all providers, and the same instructions were posted at clinic workstations for point-of-care reference. Finally, an electronic medical record (EMR) smart phrase was developed to facilitate consistent documentation of genetics referrals within clinical notes. After the protocol was implemented, we conducted Phase 2 chart reviews to extract the same variables as Phase 1.

2.2. Data Analysis

Descriptive statistics were used to summarize demographic variables as well as referral characteristics for Phase 1 and Phase 2 cohorts. Continuous variables were summarized using medians and interquartile range (IQR) and compared using the Mann-Whitney U test. Categorical variables were summarized using frequencies and percentages and compared using chi-square tests or Fisher's exact tests when expected cell counts were small. All chart review variables were complete with no missing data. Some demographic variables contained missing values; these were reported using available-case denominators in the demographic table (n and %) to reflect the number of participants with available data. Because demographic variables were not included in inferential analyses, no imputation or case exclusion procedures were necessary.

3. Results

3.1. Demographics

Chart reviews were completed on two hundred and two patients (Phase 1 $n = 88$; Phase 2 $n = 114$). Patients in Phase 1 were older on average (median = 72 months, IQR = 84.0) than those in Phase 2 (median = 54 months, IQR = 74.75), with a Mann–Whitney U test indicating a significant difference between groups ($U = 5868.5$, $p = 0.038$). See Table 1 for sample characteristics.

Approximately half of the sample was female across both phases (Phase 1: 52.3%; Phase 2: 51.8%). The racial composition was predominantly White (Phase 1: 69.9%; Phase 2: 75.7%), followed by African American patients (Phase 1: 21.7%; Phase 2: 13.1%). Further, a majority of participants identified as Hispanic (Phase 1: 55.6%; Phase 2: 73.1%).

English was the most frequently reported primary language in both phases (Phase 1: 73.6%; Phase 2: 65.5%), followed by Spanish (Phase 1: 25.3%; Phase 2: 31.9%). Public insurance was the most common insurance type in Phase 1 (52.3%), whereas private insurance was slightly more prevalent in Phase 2 (50.9%).

Regarding hearing devices, the most common device type in both phases was bilateral HA (Phase 1: 36.4%; Phase 2: 46.0%). Full demographic and clinical characteristics by phase are presented in Table 1.

https://doi.org/10.3390/children13020240

Table 1. Sample Characteristics by study phase (pre- and post-QI implementation).

	Phase 1 (Pre-QI) n = 88	Phase 2 (Post-QI) n = 114
Characteristic	**Median (*IQR*)**	**Median (*IQR*)**
Child Age (months)	72 (84)	54 (74.75)
Characteristic	***n* (%)**	***n* (%)**
Child sex		
Female	46 (52.3%)	59 (51.8%)
Male	42 (47.7%)	55 (48.2%)
Child race		
White	58 (69.9%)	81 (75.7%)
Black	18 (21.7%)	14 (13.1%)
Asian	3 (3.6%)	2 (1.9%)
More than one race	4 (4.8%)	10 (9.3%)
Child ethnicity		
Hispanic	40 (55.6%)	68 (73.1%)
Non-Hispanic	32 (44.4%)	25 (26.9%)
Devices used		
None	19 (21.6%)	17 (15%)
Hearing Aid(HA), unilateral	15 (17%)	14 (12.4%)
HA, bilateral	32 (36.4%)	52 (46%)
CI and HA, Bimodal	1 (1.1%)	7 (6.2%)
CI, unilateral	0 (0%)	2 (1.8%)
CI, bilateral	6 (6.8%)	7 (6.2%)
Bone Conduction Device (BCD), unilateral	11 (12.5%)	12 (10.6%)
BCD, bilateral	4 (4.5%)	2 (1.8%)
Primary language		
English	64 (73.6%)	74 (65.5%)
Spanish	22 (25.3%)	36 (31.9%)
Other	1 (1.1%)	3 (2.7%)
Insurance type		
None	6 (6.8%)	3 (2.6%)
Private	36 (40.9%)	58 (50.9%)
Public	46 (52.3%)	53 (46.5%)

Note. HA = hearing aid, CI = cochlear implant, BCD = bone conduction device.

3.2. Genetics Referral Outcomes by Phase

3.2.1. Referred to Genetics via Any Method

The proportion of patients with evidence of any genetics referral method differed significantly between phases. In Phase 1, 35.2% of patients had documentation of a genetics referral by any method, compared to 68.4% of patients in Phase 2. A chi-square test indicated this difference was statistically significant, $\chi^2(1, N = 202) = 22.03$, $p < 0.001$. The odds of having any genetics referral were significantly higher in Phase 2 relative to Phase 1 (OR = 3.98, 95% CI [2.21, 7.18]).

3.2.2. Referrals by Method

Significant phase differences were also observed across different methods of the genetics referral process. Specifically, whether a referral order was placed differed by phase, $\chi^2(3, N = 202) = 32.36$, $p < 0.001$. In Phase 1, 18.2% of patients had a referral order placed, compared to 46.5% in Phase 2. Similarly for documentation of a referral in the clinical note, this varied by phase with documentation present for 34.1% of Phase 1 patients versus 64.0% of Phase 2 patients [$\chi^2(3, N = 202) = 36.89$, $p < 0.001$]. Similarly, routing of clinical notes to

https://doi.org/10.3390/children13020240

the genetics team increased significantly from Phase 1 to Phase 2, $\chi^2(3, N = 202) = 32.71$, $p < 0.001$, with 5.7% of Phase 1 notes routed compared to 34.2% in Phase 2.

3.2.3. Referral Initiator

For referral order placement, the distribution of referral initiators varied by phase, $\chi^2(3, N = 202) = 32.36$, $p < 0.001$. In Phase 1, referral orders were placed exclusively by ENT providers (18.2%), with no orders initiated by audiologists or jointly. In contrast, Phase 2 demonstrated a more distributed referral pattern, with orders placed by audiologists alone (23.7%), ENT providers alone (16.7%), and jointly by audiologists and ENT/APRN providers (6.1%).

Similarly, documentation of genetics referrals in the clinical note differed significantly by phase, $\chi^2(3, N = 202) = 36.89$, $p < 0.001$. In Phase 1, documentation was most commonly completed by ENT providers (18.2%), followed by audiologists (9.1%) and joint documentation (6.8%). In Phase 2, documentation was more frequently completed by audiologists (43.0%), with additional documentation by ENT providers (7.0%) and jointly by both provider types (14.0%).

A comparable pattern was observed for the routing of clinical notes to the genetics team, $\chi^2(3, N = 202) = 32.71$, $p < 0.001$. In Phase 1, routed notes were initiated only by ENT providers (5.7%). In Phase 2, note routing occurred primarily through audiologists (28.1%), with additional contributions from ENT providers (3.5%) and joint routing by both provider types (2.6%).

3.3. *Genetics Appointment Completion and Testing Outcomes*

Genetics appointment outcomes differed significantly by phase [$\chi^2(3, N = 202) = 39.79$, $p < 0.001$]. In Phase 1, 11.4% of patients completed a genetics appointment, whereas 38.6% of patients in Phase 2 completed an appointment.

Additionally, number of patients identified with a genetic mutation were significantly different between phases with 4.6% of patients identified in Phase 1 compared to 28.2% of patients in Phase 2 [$\chi^2(3, N = 201) = 34.92$, $p < 0.001$].

4. Discussion

In this QI initiative, implementation of a standardized, clinic-wide genetics referral protocol was associated with significant improvements across multiple points in the referral pathway, including documentation, referral order placement, appointment completion, and identification of genetic etiologies for hearing loss.

Within our large, multi-ethnic university-based multidisciplinary audiology and otolaryngology practice, with integrated genetic support, the proportion of patients with a documented genetics referral nearly doubled, completion of a genetics appointment increased more than threefold, and identification of genetic etiology for hearing loss increased significantly. Collectively, these findings suggest that targeted workflow standardization can significantly improve access to and completion of genetic evaluation in pediatric hearing loss without requiring additional institutional resources.

Genetic testing plays a critical role in the evaluation of pediatric hearing loss by informing etiology, prognosis, genetic counseling, and timing of intervention, all of which directly influence clinical outcomes. Identification of a genetic etiology can guide anticipatory guidance, surveillance, and multidisciplinary care for associated syndromic conditions, including Usher syndrome, Pendred syndrome, Alport syndrome, and Jervell and Lange-Nielsen syndrome. Improving access to genetic evaluation may reduce diagnostic uncertainty, support family counseling regarding recurrence risk, and improve coordination of care across specialties.

https://doi.org/10.3390/children13020240

This initiative aligns with core QI principles by addressing workflow barriers through standardized process redesign and iterative provider education. Prior to implementation, variability in referral practices likely reflected uncertainty regarding responsibility, timing, and expectations. The QI initiative appears to have improved outcomes by clarifying the referral pathway and reducing reliance on individual provider discretion. Audiologists demonstrated the greatest improvement in referral initiation and documentation, which is clinically important given that they are often the first providers to confirm permanent hearing loss and initiate diagnostic evaluation. Empowering audiologists to initiate and document genetics referrals reduced dependence on downstream provider action and facilitated earlier engagement of genetics services. These findings underscore the importance of shared responsibility within multidisciplinary hearing loss care teams and highlight audiologists as key drivers of timely, guideline concordant genetic evaluation.

This intervention was designed to be sustainable within routine clinical practice. The use of EMR smart phrases, point-of-care reminders, and standardized documentation requires minimal ongoing maintenance and does not rely on additional personnel or clinic time. Implementation in a racially, ethnically, and linguistically diverse pediatric population also suggests that standardized workflows may promote more equitable access to genetic services by mitigating variability related to language barriers, insurance status, or differences in provider counseling practices. These features support long-term sustainability and facilitate adoption of similar workflows in other pediatric audiology and otolaryngology settings.

A modest difference in mean age was observed between Phase 1 and Phase 2, with children in Phase 2 being somewhat younger on average. Although age could theoretically influence referral practices, current pediatric hearing loss guidelines recommend etiologic and genetic evaluation for all children with permanent hearing loss irrespective of age at diagnosis. Therefore, this difference was unlikely to fully explain the observed increase in referrals following protocol implementation.

Prior research consistently demonstrates gaps between guideline recommendations for genetic evaluation and actual clinical practice in pediatric hearing loss. Both the American College of Medical Genetics and Genomics (ACMG) and the Joint Committee on Infant Hearing (JCIH) recommend genetic evaluation as part of the diagnostic workup for children with permanent hearing loss to improve etiologic diagnosis, counseling, and management [6,19]. Despite these recommendations, multiple studies have documented low rates of genetics referral and testing in routine care [20]. QI initiatives in other clinical populations have demonstrated that structured workflow interventions, such as standardized referral tools, provider education, and integration of genetics services into clinical workflows, can significantly improve referral and completion rates for genetic counseling and testing [21,22]. In contrast to resource-intensive models, the standardized referral workflow implemented in the present initiative improved referral and completion outcomes without requiring additional specialized resources.

Limitations of this study should be acknowledged. This study used a retrospective, non-randomized pre–post design as part of a quality improvement initiative; therefore, causal inferences regarding the effect of the intervention should be interpreted cautiously, as system-level factors may also have influenced outcomes. Although referral outcomes were defined a priori and reflected distinct steps in the clinical workflow, multiple related comparisons were conducted without formal adjustment for multiplicity, consistent with the descriptive and process-focused nature of QI evaluations. In addition, this was a retrospective, single-institution initiative, which may limit generalizability. Genetic testing performed outside our institution was excluded to maintain focus on referral practices within our clinical workflow; this exclusion may result in underestimation of overall

https://doi.org/10.3390/children13020240

genetic testing rates. Additionally, retrospective chart review is inherently limited by incomplete documentation. Nevertheless, improving documentation accuracy remains a critical component of effective care coordination and continuity. Finally, the study timeframe limited assessment of long-term patient outcomes, including the downstream clinical impact of earlier genetic diagnosis.

5. Conclusions

Implementation of a standardized referral protocol for genetic evaluation in pediatric hearing loss significantly improved referral rates, the completion of genetic appointments, and the identification of genetic etiologies in our cohort. This QI initiative demonstrates that low-cost, standardized workflow implementation can significantly improve adherence to guideline recommended care for pediatric hearing loss. The adoption of similar referral standardization and provider training may help close the gap between evidence-based recommendations for genetic testing and clinical practice in pediatric ENT care. Future work should evaluate the sustainability of this intervention over time, assess patient-centered outcomes, and explore implementation across diverse clinical settings to further advance equitable, guideline concordant care for children with hearing loss.

Author Contributions: Conceptualization, J.C., C.M.S., I.C., and X.Z.L.; Methodology, J.C., C.M.S., I.C., V.Y., and X.Z.L.; Validation, J.C., C.M.S., I.C., V.Y., and J.A.M.; Formal Analysis, J.C., I.C., and V.Y.; Investigation, J.C., C.M.S., I.C., V.Y., J.A.M., and X.Z.L.; Data Curation, J.C., V.Y., and I.C.; Writing—Original Draft Preparation, J.C., I.C., J.A.M., V.Y., and C.M.S.; Writing—Review and Editing, J.C., I.C., and X.Z.L.; Visualization, J.C. and I.C.; Funding Acquisition, I.C. and X.Z.L. All authors have read and agreed to the published version of the manuscript.

Funding: This project was supported in part by NIDCD R25 DC020726 to Xue-Zhong Liu. Dr. Liu's lab is supported by NIH grants of R01DC022239, R01DC005575, R01DC107624, and RH220053-W81XWH-22-HRRP-FRA.

Institutional Review Board Statement: The study was conducted in accordance with the Declaration of Helsinki and approved by the Institutional Review Board (or Ethics Committee) of University of Miami (protocol 20230863, date of approval: 29 August 2023).

Informed Consent Statement: Informed consent was waived by the IRB given the retrospective nature of the study.

Data Availability Statement: The original contributions presented in this study are included in the article. Further inquiries can be directed to the corresponding author.

Conflicts of Interest: C.M.S.—Cochlear research grant; J.C.—MED-EL research grant; V.Y.—none; J.M.—none; I.C.—Cochlear, Regeneron, NIH research grants, consultant for Regeneron, Advanced Bionics, and Cochlear; X.L.—NIH research grants. The conflicts of interest had no role in the design of the study; in the collection, analyses, or interpretation of data; in the writing of the manuscript; or in the decision to publish the results.

References

1. World Health Organization. Deafness and Hearing Loss. Available online: https://www.who.int/news-room/fact-sheets/detail/deafness-and-hearing-loss (accessed on 22 January 2026).
2. Korver, A.M.H.; Smith, R.J.H.; Van Camp, G.; Schleiss, M.R.; Bitner-Glindzicz, M.A.K.; Lustig, L.R.; Usami, S.; Boudewyns, A.N. Congenital Hearing Loss. *Nat. Rev. Dis. Primers* **2017**, *3*, 16094. [CrossRef] [PubMed]
3. National Institute on Deafness and Other Communication Disorders (NIDCD). Quick Statistics About Hearing, Balance, & Dizziness. Available online: https://www.nidcd.nih.gov/health/statistics/quick-statistics-hearing (accessed on 22 January 2026).
4. Lee, N.K.; Uhler, K.M.; Yoon, P.J.; Santos-Cortez, R.L.P. Clinical Genetic Testing for Hearing Loss: Implications for Genetic Counseling and Gene-Based Therapies. *Biomedicines* **2024**, *12*, 1427. [CrossRef] [PubMed]

5. Božanić Urbančič, N.; Battelino, S.; Tesovnik, T.; Trebušak Podkrajšek, K. The Importance of Early Genetic Diagnostics of Hearing Loss in Children. *Medicina* **2020**, *56*, 471. [CrossRef] [PubMed]
6. Alford, R.L.; Arnos, K.S.; Fox, M.; Lin, J.W.; Palmer, C.G.; Pandya, A.; Rehm, H.L.; Robin, N.H.; Scott, D.A.; Yoshinaga-Itano, C. American College of Medical Genetics and Genomics Guideline for the Clinical Evaluation and Etiologic Diagnosis of Hearing Loss. *Genet. Med.* **2014**, *16*, 347–355. [CrossRef] [PubMed]
7. Zhong, L.X.; Kun, S.; Jing, Q.; Jing, C.; Denise, Y. Non-Syndromic Hearing Loss and High-Throughput Strategies to Decipher Its Genetic Heterogeneity. *J. Otol.* **2013**, *8*, 6–24. [CrossRef]
8. Moeller, M.P.; Tomblin, J.B.; Yoshinaga-Itano, C.; Connor, C.M.; Jerger, S. Current State of Knowledge: Language and Literacy of Children with Hearing Impairment. *Ear Hear.* **2007**, *28*, 740. [CrossRef] [PubMed]
9. Ching, T.Y.C. Is Early Intervention Effective in Improving Spoken Language Outcomes of Children With Congenital Hearing Loss? *Am. J. Audiol.* **2015**, *24*, 345–348. [CrossRef] [PubMed]
10. Stika, C.J.; Eisenberg, L.S.; Johnson, K.C.; Henning, S.C.; Colson, B.G.; Ganguly, D.H.; DesJardin, J.L. Developmental Outcomes of Early-Identified Children Who Are Hard of Hearing at 12 to 18months of Age. *Early Hum. Dev.* **2015**, *91*, 47–55. [CrossRef] [PubMed]
11. Han, J.H.; Kim, S.H.; Moon, I.S.; Joo, S.Y.; Kim, J.A.; Gee, H.Y.; Jung, J.; Choi, J.Y. Comprehensive Prediction Model, Including Genetic Testing, for the Outcomes of Cochlear Implantation. *Ear Hear.* **2023**, *44*, 223–231. [CrossRef] [PubMed]
12. Ismail, N.M.; Galal, S.B.; Behairy, R.M.; Sabry, R.M. Systematic Review of Outcomes of Cochlear Implantation of Different Genotypes in Patients with Auditory Neuropathy Spectrum Disorder. *Egypt. J. Otolaryngol.* **2024**, *40*, 102. [CrossRef]
13. Xiang, J.; Jin, Y.; Song, N.; Chen, S.; Shen, J.; Xie, W.; Sun, X.; Peng, Z.; Sun, Y. Comprehensive Genetic Testing Improves the Clinical Diagnosis and Medical Management of Pediatric Patients with Isolated Hearing Loss. *BMC Med. Genom.* **2022**, *15*, 142. [CrossRef] [PubMed]
14. Barnett, C.L.; Malhotra, P.; VanHorn, A.; Zaharieva, B.; Myers, J.; Riggs, W.J.; Jordan, E. Utilization of Genetics Services in the Diagnosis of Hearing Loss in Newborns in the State of Ohio. *J. Community Genet.* **2025**, *16*, 603–613. [CrossRef] [PubMed]
15. Robin, N.H.; Prucka, S.K.; Woolley, A.L.; Smith, R.J. The Use of Genetic Testing in the Evaluation of Hearing Impairment in a Child. *Curr. Opin. Pediatr.* **2005**, *17*, 709–712. [CrossRef] [PubMed]
16. Gooch, C.; Rudy, N.; Smith, R.J.H.; Robin, N.H. Genetic Testing Hearing Loss: The Challenge of Non Syndromic Mimics. *Int. J. Pediatr. Otorhinolaryngol.* **2021**, *150*, 110872. [CrossRef] [PubMed]
17. Yan, D.; Tekin, M.; Blanton, S.H.; Liu, X.Z. Next-Generation Sequencing in Genetic Hearing Loss. *Genet. Test. Mol. Biomark.* **2013**, *17*, 581–587. [CrossRef]
18. Cejas, I.; Coto, J.; Sarangoulis, C.M.; Yunis, V.; Blanton, S.; Liu, X.Z. Parent Experiences with Genetic Testing for Pediatric Hearing Loss. *J. Genet. Couns.* **2025**, *34*, e1986. [CrossRef] [PubMed]
19. Joint Committee on Infant Hearing. Year 2019 Position Statement: Principles and Guidelines for Early Hearing Detection and Intervention Programs. *J. Early Hear. Detect. Interv.* **2019**, *4*, 1–44.
20. Bush, M.L.; Hardin, B.; Rayle, C.; Lester, C.; Studts, C.R.; Shinn, J.B. Rural Barriers to Early Diagnosis and Treatment of Infant Hearing Loss in Appalachia. *Otol. Neurotol.* **2015**, *36*, 93–98. [CrossRef] [PubMed]
21. Plaskocinska, I.; Shipman, H.; Drummond, J.; Thompson, E.; Buchanan, V.; Newcombe, B.; Hodgkin, C.; Barter, E.; Ridley, P.; Ng, R.; et al. New Paradigms for BRCA1/BRCA2 Testing in Women with Ovarian Cancer: Results of the Genetic Testing in Epithelial Ovarian Cancer (GTEOC) Study. *J. Med. Genet.* **2016**, *53*, 655–661. [CrossRef] [PubMed]
22. Swanson, C.L.; Kumar, A.; Maharaj, J.M.; Kemppainen, J.L.; Thomas, B.C.; Weinhold, M.R.; Slaby, K.M.; Mara, K.C.; Wick, M.J.; Bakkum-Gamez, J.N. Increasing Genetic Counseling Referral Rates through Bundled Interventions after Ovarian Cancer Diagnosis. *Gynecol. Oncol.* **2018**, *149*, 121–126. [CrossRef] [PubMed]

https://doi.org/10.3390/children13020240

children

MDPI

Article

Follow-Up of Hearing Impairment in Patients with Congenital CMV Infection

Ron Fisher [1,*], Miriam Geal Dor [2,3], Cahtia Adelman [2,3], Michal Kaufmann-Yehezkely [1] and Sagit Stern Shavit [1]

1 Department of Otolaryngology-Head and Neck Surgery, Hadassah Medical Center, Faculty of Medicine, Hebrew University of Jerusalem, Jerusalem 9112102, Israel; dkau375@hadassah.org.il (M.K.-Y.); sagitst@dom.hadassah.org.il (S.S.S.)
2 Speech & Hearing Center, Hadassah Medical Center, Hebrew University of Jerusalem, Jerusalem 9112102, Israel; gmiriam@hadassah.org.il (M.G.D.); cahtiaa@hadassah.org.il (C.A.)
3 Department of Communication Disorders, Jerusalem Multidisciplinary College, Jerusalem 9422408, Israel
* Correspondence: ronf@hadassah.org.il

Highlights

What are the main findings?

- Delayed-onset SNHL in children with congenital CMV frequently develops after an initial period of normal hearing and may present over a broad age range.
- While poorer-ear thresholds are comparable, better-ear hearing remains more preserved in delayed-onset SNHL compared with congenital SNHL.

What are the implications of the main findings?

- cCMV-related hearing loss follows heterogeneous and asymmetric trajectories, with dynamic changes and progression in a substantial proportion of children.
- Detection and characterization of SNHL in cCMV depend on prolonged follow-up, underscoring both its clinical value and practical challenges.

Abstract

Background/Objectives: Congenital cytomegalovirus (cCMV) is a leading non-genetic cause of childhood sensorineural hearing loss (SNHL), characterized by heterogeneous and dynamic hearing outcomes. Hearing impairment may be present at birth or emerge later in childhood. This study aimed to characterize hearing trajectories and laterality patterns in children with cCMV, with emphasis on congenital versus delayed-onset SNHL. **Methods**: We conducted a retrospective study of children with confirmed cCMV who underwent longitudinal audiologic follow-up. Hearing loss was classified as congenital SNHL or delayed-onset SNHL. Better- and poorer-ear thresholds, bilateral involvement, longitudinal changes, and follow-up duration were analyzed. **Results**: Of 195 included children, 59 (30%) developed SNHL. Congenital SNHL was present in 34 children (17%), while delayed-onset SNHL developed in 25 of 161 children (16%) who were born with normal hearing. Of these delayed-onset cases, 20 (80%) were asymptomatic at birth, while 5 (20%) presented with non-audiological neonatal symptoms. Longitudinal observation of the delayed-onset subgroup revealed that 36 ears developed SNHL during follow-up, spanning infancy through later childhood, including one case identified in early adulthood. Better-ear thresholds were significantly better preserved in delayed-onset SNHL, while poorer-ear thresholds were comparable across groups. Children with SNHL had substantially longer follow-up duration (60 ± 44.5 months) compared with those with normal hearing (37 ± 24.4 months). **Conclusions**: Children with cCMV-related SNHL exhibit dynamic and asymmetric hearing trajectories with clinically relevant differences between congenital and delayed-onset SNHL. These findings underscore the necessity of a risk-stratified, long-term surveillance framework that ensures individualized long-term monitoring and promotes sustained adherence to follow-up.

Keywords: congenital CMV; follow-up; hearing monitoring; delayed-onset SNHL; progressive hearing loss

1. Introduction

Cytomegalovirus (CMV), a member of the *Herpesviridae* family, is the most common cause of congenital infection worldwide. The incidence of congenital cytomegalovirus (cCMV) varies globally, ranging from 0.2% to 2.0% of live births, with an average of 0.64% [1]. In Israel, the prevalence is estimated at approximately 0.7% [2].

Although most infected newborns are asymptomatic, cCMV is a leading cause of childhood sensorineural hearing loss (SNHL), accounting for about a quarter of all cases of hearing loss by age 4 years [3]. The clinical spectrum of cCMV is broad and heterogeneous. While 10–15% of newborns are symptomatic at birth—with up to half of them developing SNHL—the vast majority (85–90%) appear asymptomatic. Crucially, approximately 10–15% of these initially asymptomatic infants, who pass their newborn hearing screening, will still develop delayed-onset SNHL later in childhood [1,4–6], with lower rates reported in some large registry-based cohorts [7]. This distinction between congenital and postnatal manifestations is critical, as it underscores a prolonged window of vulnerability for the auditory system.

The biological mechanisms underlying CMV-related auditory damage remain incompletely understood [8]. Current evidence suggests that delayed-onset symptoms may arise from the reactivation of latent virus within the spiral ganglion or scala media [9]. Additionally, chronic inflammatory processes in the stria vascularis, characterized by persistent cytokine release, and progressive neural degeneration secondary to subclinical early viral injury have been proposed as key drivers of late-onset SNHL [10,11]. Together, these processes contribute to the unpredictable timing and progression of hearing loss, thereby justifying prolonged longitudinal audiologic surveillance in children with cCMV.

The risk of SNHL is influenced by maternal, viral, and neonatal factors. Regarding maternal infection, both the nature and timing of infection during gestation are critical. Primary maternal infection confers a substantially higher vertical transmission rate (approx. 30–40%) than non-primary infection (1–2%) [6,12]. Importantly, while the rate of vertical transmission increases as gestation progresses, the risk of severe fetal sequelae, including SNHL, is highest during the first trimester (approximately 22.8%) and decreases significantly when transmission occurs in the second or third trimesters [13].

Following transmission, the neonate's clinical status serves as a key prognostic indicator. Several neonatal factors are associated with an increased risk of SNHL, including symptomatic disease at birth—characterized by findings such as petechiae, thrombocytopenia, hepatosplenomegaly or elevated liver enzymes [14], as well as high neonatal viral load [15] and neuroimaging abnormalities such as ventriculomegaly and white matter abnormalities [7,16].

Because early identification and intervention are critical for speech, language, and neurodevelopment, frequent repeated auditory monitoring for children with cCMV is essential [10]. However, existing guidelines differ in both the frequency and duration of follow-up, with recommendations ranging from surveillance until age 3–6 years [17,18]

https://doi.org/10.3390/children13020230

to continued monitoring into adolescence or adulthood [6,19]. Evidence supporting these extended schedules remains limited, and the optimal duration and intensity of surveillance remain unknown.

To address these gaps, this study aims to characterize long-term hearing trajectories and patterns of onset and progression in children with cCMV, while also evaluating real-world adherence to prolonged audiologic follow-up—key factors for informing evidence-based surveillance strategies.

2. Materials and Methods

We conducted a retrospective cohort study of children with cCMV born between the years 2005–2019 who were followed at Hadassah Medical Center between 2005 and 2025. Inclusion criteria were: (1) confirmed diagnosis of cCMV; (2) at least 4 documented audiologic assessments; and (3) follow-up period exceeding 1 year. The requirement for at least four assessments was used to ensure reliable longitudinal data within a single institution and to minimize loss of follow-up information. Diagnosis of cCMV infection was established by detection of CMV-DNA using polymerase chain reaction (PCR) in neonatal urine samples obtained within the first three weeks of life. We excluded children with known genetic causes of hearing loss or alternative clear etiologies for SNHL (e.g., meningitis, ototoxic chemotherapy), craniofacial anomalies, chronic inflammatory middle-ear disease, or those with incomplete audiologic data.

Clinical data were extracted from electronic medical records, and included birth weight, gestational age, neonatal intensive care unit (NICU) admission, neurologic signs, neuroimaging abnormalities, jaundice or hepatitis, thrombocytopenia, petechiae, pulmonary or ophthalmologic findings, and administration of antiviral therapy. Antiviral treatment (valganciclovir) was administered by a pediatric infectious disease specialist in children with cCMV-related systemic symptoms and/or sensorineural hearing loss.

2.1. Hearing Assessment

Audiological evaluations included both objective and behavioral tests. Initial objective assessments consisted of Transient Evoked Otoacoustic Emissions (TEOAE) and Automated Auditory Brainstem Response (AABR) performed prior to hospital discharge using Otodynamics system (Echocheck and Otoport; Otodynamics Ltd., Hatfield, UK).

At our institution, infants with confirmed cCMV follow a structured surveillance protocol. This includes an initial diagnostic ABR evaluation in early infancy, followed by audiologic monitoring every 3 months up to 18 months of age, every 6 months up to 3 years, and annually thereafter until age 7.

Diagnostic ABR thresholds were obtained in young infants using a Biologic Navigator-Pro Evoked Potential System (Natus Medical Inc., Mundelein, IL, USA) or an Interacoustics Eclipse system (Interacoustics, Middelfart, Denmark). Threshold was obtained in response to alternating stimuli, presented at a rate of 21.1 stimuli per second for click, and 39 stimuli per second for tonal stimuli at 1 kHz and 4 kHz. The stimuli consisted of at least 1024 sweeps with filter settings of 30–3000 Hz for clicks and 30–1500 Hz for tone bursts, using insert earphones and bone conduction as needed.

Behavioral assessments included visual reinforcement audiometry (VRA) for speech and tonal stimuli between 7 and 24 months, using insert earphones and bone conduction as needed. From approximately 2–3 years of age, conditioned play audiometry (CPA) and speech reception thresholds (SRTs) were obtained with a clinical audiometer (Interacoustics AC40, Assens, Denmark). When behavioral responses were unreliable or insufficient, sedated ABR was performed. Tympanometry was routinely used to assess middle-ear status.

https://doi.org/10.3390/children13020230

Hearing impairment was classified by type (sensorineural or conductive), laterality (unilateral or bilateral), and severity: mild (20–40 dB), moderate (41–70 dB), severe (71–90 dB), or profound (>91 dB). Based on hearing status at birth and during follow-up, children were categorized as having congenital SNHL, delayed-onset SNHL, or normal hearing. Longitudinal hearing status was categorized as stable or deteriorated. Conductive hearing loss (CHL) was documented during follow-up. Children with isolated CHL were excluded from SNHL outcome analyses and grouped with children without SNHL for descriptive analyses, as the study focused on cCMV-related sensorineural hearing loss.

2.2. Statistical Analysis

Categorical variables are presented as counts and percentages and were compared using the chi-square test or Fisher's exact test as appropriate. Pure-tone and ABR thresholds were treated as non-normally distributed and compared using the Mann–Whitney U test for both within-group (better vs. poorer ear) and between-group (congenital vs. delayed-onset SNHL) comparisons. Hearing thresholds and laterality were compared between treated and untreated children within the SNHL subgroup using the Mann–Whitney U and Fisher's exact tests. The timing of delayed-onset SNHL was evaluated by plotting the cumulative number of newly diagnosed ears as a function of age at first detection. Each affected ear was included once, at the age when SNHL was initially identified. This analysis was used to describe the temporal distribution of delayed-onset SNHL across the follow-up period. Odds ratios (ORs) with 95% confidence intervals (CIs) were calculated for selected comparisons. Two-sided p-values < 0.05 were considered statistically significant. All statistical analyses were performed with GraphPad Prism 10.6.1.

3. Results

A total of 800 infants with cCMV were identified in our database. Of these, 198 met the inclusion criteria of having ≥4 documented audiologic assessments over more than one year of follow-up. Three children were excluded due to meningitis, hereditary immune disorder, and ototoxic chemotherapy, leaving a final cohort of 195 children.

Overall, 59 children (30%) developed SNHL. Among these, 34 (58%) had congenital SNHL and 25 (42%) developed delayed-onset SNHL. The remaining 136 children (70%) maintained normal hearing or only mild conductive hearing loss throughout follow-up. Among children with congenital SNHL, 21 (62%) remained stable, whereas 13 (38%) demonstrated progressive deterioration (Figure 1).

Average follow-up duration was 43.5 ± 33.5 months and extended beyond five years in 25% of children, between two and five years in 43%, and between one and two years in 32%.

Table 1 summarizes baseline characteristics across the three hearing-outcome groups (Congenital SNHL, Delayed-Onset SNHL, and Normal Hearing). Non-audiologic cCMV manifestations at birth (symptomatic cCMV infection) were documented in 52 of 195 (26.7%) infants and differed significantly between hearing-outcome groups ($p = 0.00012$). All children in the study underwent cranial ultrasound (US) after birth to screen for intracranial abnormalities. Of these, 43 children had abnormal neuroimaging findings; the most frequent were subependymal cysts (n = 18), followed by intracranial calcifications (n = 9), ventriculomegaly (n = 7), and microcephaly (n = 5). An additional 10 children exhibited other non-specific neuroimaging findings and developmental delay. Neurologic abnormalities were more common in the congenital SNHL group compared with the delayed-onset or the normal-hearing groups (47% vs. 20% and 16%, respectively; $p = 0.00051$). Jaundice and elevated liver enzymes showed a similar gradient, being substantially more frequent among infants with congenital SNHL (15% vs. 4% and 1.5%, respectively; $p = 0.00234$).

https://doi.org/10.3390/children13020230

Other birth findings were infrequent and did not differ significantly, although several trended higher in children with congenital SNHL.

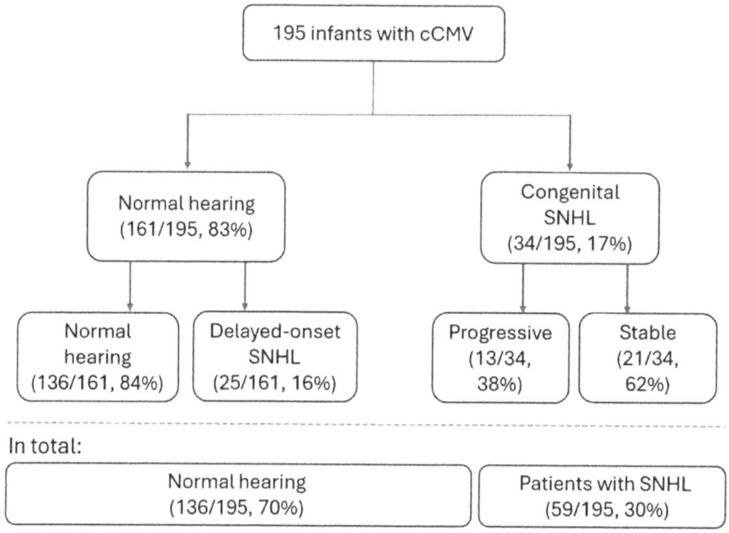

Figure 1. Flow diagram of hearing outcomes in children with congenital cytomegalovirus infection. Children were categorized according to hearing status at birth and during follow-up. Numbers indicate counts and percentages relative to the total cohort (n = 195).

Table 1. Baseline demographic and clinical characteristics of infants with congenital CMV, stratified by hearing outcome. Values are presented as n (%). *p*-values reflect comparisons across the three hearing outcome groups using the chi-square test. For antiviral treatment, Fisher's exact test was used to compare the congenital SNHL and delayed-onset SNHL groups only. Abbreviations—SNHL, sensorineural hearing loss; IUGR, intrauterine growth restriction. * Statistically significant ($p < 0.05$).

Characteristic	Total (n = 195)	Congenital SNHL (n = 34)	Delayed-Onset SNHL (n = 25)	Normal Hearing (n = 136)	*p*-Value
Female	84 (43%)	17 (50%)	9 (36%)	58 (43%)	0.553
Antiviral treatment	56 (29%)	22 (65%)	9 (36%)	25 (18%)	0.037 *
Non-audiological symptoms at birth (Symptomatic at birth)	52 (27%)	19 (56%)	5 (20%)	28 (21%)	0.00012 *
Neurological findings	43 (22%)	16 (47%)	5 (20%)	22 (16%)	0.00051 *
Dermatological findings	2 (1%)	1 (3%)	1 (4%)	0 (0%)	0.090
Ocular findings	4 (2%)	2 (6%)	0 (0%)	2 (1%)	0.198
Jaundice/elevated liver enzymes	8 (4%)	5 (15%)	1 (4%)	2 (1%)	0.00234 *
Hematological abnormalities	12 (6%)	5 (15%)	1 (4%)	6 (4%)	0.073
Respiratory findings	6 (3%)	0 (0%)	0 (0%)	6 (4%)	0.261
IUGR	11 (6%)	3 (9%)	1 (4%)	7 (5%)	0.658
Prematurity (<37 wk)	21 (11%)	3 (9%)	0 (0%)	18 (13%)	0.135

https://doi.org/10.3390/children13020230

Antiviral therapy was administered to 56 of 195 children (29%). Treatment was significantly more common in the congenital SNHL group (22/34, 65%) than in the delayed-onset SNHL group (9/25, 36%) or the normal hearing group (25/136, 18%; $p = 0.037$). However, statistical comparison revealed no significant differences in final hearing thresholds between treated and untreated children for either the poorer ear ($p = 0.7015$) or the better ear ($p = 0.1628$). Additionally, the proportion of bilateral versus unilateral SNHL was not significantly different between the groups ($p = 0.0692$).

Age at last audiologic assessment differed significantly by hearing outcome. Children with normal hearing had their last evaluation at a mean age of 37 ± 24.4 months, whereas children with SNHL (congenital or delayed-onset) were followed longer (mean 60 ± 44.5 months, mean difference 23 months, 95% CI 10.7–35.3; $p = 0.0004$).

Bilateral hearing involvement was present in 30 of 59 children (51%) with SNHL, 59% in the congenital SNHL group and 44% in the delayed-onset SNHL group ($p = 0.192$; OR 1.82, 95% CI 0.64–5.16).

Hearing thresholds were analyzed separately for the better and poorer ear, as only a minority of the children demonstrated symmetric loss. Figure 2 shows individual thresholds for congenital and delayed-onset SNHL. In both groups, the poorer-ear median threshold was 90 dB (IQR 70–100 dB). In contrast, better-ear thresholds differed significantly between groups, with median values of 30 dB (IQR 17.5–82.5 dB) in congenital SNHL and 15 dB (IQR 10–38.8 dB) in delayed-onset SNHL ($p = 0.0146$).

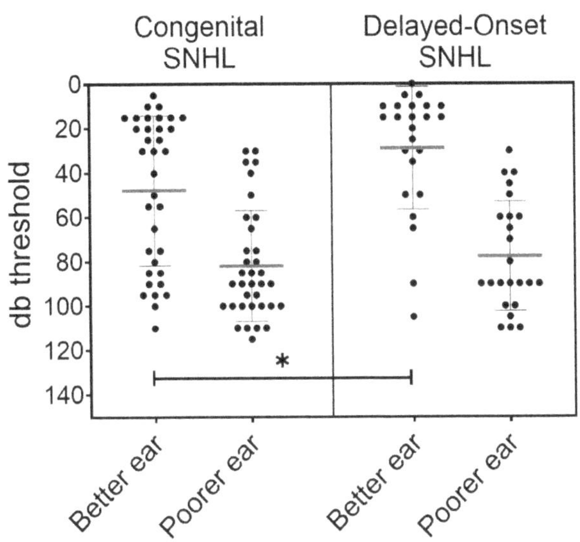

Figure 2. Better- and poorer-ear pure-tone thresholds in congenital and delayed-onset cCMV-related hearing loss. Individual ear thresholds are shown as scatter plots, grouped by clinical phenotype (**left**: congenital SNHL; **right**: delayed-onset SNHL) and by better versus poorer ear. Red horizontal lines represent group medians, and grey whiskers denote interquartile ranges. Within each group, poorer-ear thresholds were significantly higher than better-ear thresholds (Mann–Whitney, $p < 0.05$). Across groups, better-ear thresholds were significantly worse in the congenital SNHL group compared with the delayed-onset group ($p = 0.0146$), whereas poorer-ear thresholds did not differ between groups. * Indicates a statistically significant difference ($p < 0.05$).

Timing of delayed-onset SNHL varied widely. Among the 25 children with delayed-onset SNHL, hearing loss developed in 37 of 50 ears (74%) during follow-up. Most diagnoses occurred early in life, with over half identified by two years of age. A further

https://doi.org/10.3390/children13020230

proportion was diagnosed between two and five years, and two ears (5%) were diagnosed after the age of five, including one case identified in adulthood (20 years). In these cases, a comprehensive diagnostic work-up was performed to rule-out alternative causes of SNHL. The cumulative distribution of age at first detection is shown in Figure 3.

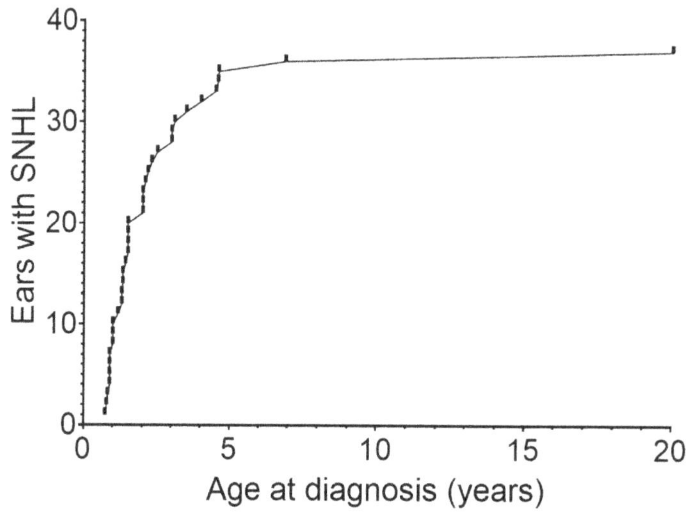

Figure 3. Cumulative number of ears diagnosed with delayed-onset SNHL by age at first detection. The curve depicts the cumulative count of ears in which delayed-onset SNHL was first identified during follow-up. Each increase represents a newly diagnosed ear at the corresponding age.

4. Discussion

Congenital cytomegalovirus (cCMV) is a well-recognized cause of childhood sensorineural hearing loss (SNHL), yet the timing and progression of auditory impairment remain highly variable. The prevalence of SNHL in our cohort (30%) is consistent with previously reported rates ranging from 20% to 40% in both population-based and referral cohorts [5,20,21]. As described in prior studies, hearing loss was not confined to the neonatal period and could emerge or progress over time, including in children who initially passed newborn hearing screening.

We observed a relatively high proportion of symptomatic cases in our cohort (27%), exceeding the 10–15% typically reported in the literature [17,22]. This likely reflects the retrospective design and follow-up related selection bias, as children with early symptoms or clinical concerns are more likely to remain under longitudinal surveillance. Since April 2022, universal newborn cCMV screening has been implemented at our institution with structured audiologic follow-up [23], and future analyses of this prospective cohort are expected to provide a more representative estimate of symptom prevalence and long-term hearing trajectories.

Delayed-onset SNHL occurred in 16% of children with initially normal hearing, consistent with earlier reports describing delayed hearing loss in 10–15% of asymptomatic or mildly symptomatic infants with cCMV [5,21]. Although a recent large-scale European registry reported a lower incidence [7], this difference likely reflects variations in study design, follow-up duration, and surveillance intensity. In our cohort, most delayed-onset cases were identified within the first few years of life; however, a small number were diagnosed after the age at which routine follow-up is often discontinued. The frequent fluctuations and deteriorations observed in affected children, together with the occurrence

https://doi.org/10.3390/children13020230

of late-onset SNHL, underscore the prolonged and unpredictable risk window associated with cCMV-related hearing loss.

Delayed-onset and progressive SNHL in cCMV are increasingly understood as manifestations of ongoing pathological processes rather than static neonatal injury. Proposed mechanisms include reactivation of latent virus within the spiral ganglion or scala media, chronic or recurrent inflammatory activity within the stria vascularis, and progressive cochlear or neural degeneration following subclinical early viral injury [4,9–11]. These mechanisms provide a biological framework for the variable timing and progression observed in our cohort and support the rationale for longitudinal audiologic surveillance.

Analysis of ear-specific hearing thresholds demonstrated that poorer-ear thresholds reached comparable severity in both congenital and delayed-onset SNHL, whereas better-ear thresholds were more preserved in children with delayed-onset loss. This finding aligns with previous reports emphasizing asymmetric progression and earlier deterioration of the poorer-hearing ear in cCMV-associated SNHL [24]. Our data suggest that delayed-onset SNHL often follows a milder and more asymmetric course, while congenital SNHL more frequently involves bilateral and progressive disease, as reported in earlier cohorts [22,25].

Bilateral involvement was observed in 51% (30/59) of children with SNHL and in 59% of those with congenital SNHL, closely matching the 60–65% rates reported in systematic reviews of cCMV-associated congenital hearing loss [4]. Nearly half of children with congenital SNHL (47%) presented with severe-to-profound hearing loss at diagnosis, and 38% demonstrated progressive or fluctuating hearing thresholds over time, consistent with the 30–35% frequency of dynamic hearing patterns described in previous studies [5].

In our cohort, antiviral therapy was not significantly associated with final hearing outcomes within the SNHL subgroups. However, these findings should be interpreted with caution due to the non-randomized, retrospective nature of the study, where treatment was clinically indicated based on diverse symptoms and onset patterns.

A major clinical finding of this study relates to long-term follow-up adherence and its implications for surveillance strategies in children with cCMV. Nearly one-third of children discontinued audiologic follow-up within the first two years of life, most commonly those without early hearing impairment who nonetheless remain at risk for delayed-onset SNHL. Similar challenges have been reported in other cohorts and reflect real-world barriers to prolonged monitoring, including logistical, socioeconomic, and family-related factors [26–28].

At our institution, structured audiologic surveillance is conducted up to seven years of age; however, our findings demonstrate that hearing loss onset spans a broad age range, including cases identified beyond the period typically covered by routine follow-up programs. These observations highlight the need to balance the clinical benefit of early detection against the economic and practical burden of long-term surveillance. Rather than a rigid one-size-fits-all protocol, follow-up may benefit from a risk-stratified, family-centered approach that considers factors such as the trimester of maternal infection, primary versus non-primary infection status, neonatal symptom status, initial hearing thresholds, and the presence of language, motor, or vestibular deficits [5,16,26]. At the same time, our data demonstrate that delayed-onset SNHL can also occur in children initially considered low risk, underscoring the potential for missed diagnoses if surveillance is prematurely reduced. Long-term observational data, such as those presented here, together with future prospective studies and expert consensus, are therefore essential to define evidence-based, sustainable monitoring frameworks.

Vestibular findings were beyond the scope of the data available in this retrospective cohort, as standardized vestibular testing was not routinely performed. Nevertheless, vestibular dysfunction is increasingly recognized as a common and clinically significant manifestation of cCMV, with important implications for balance, motor development, and

https://doi.org/10.3390/children13020230

overall neurodevelopment, and it may occur independently of hearing status. Recent studies have highlighted the high prevalence of vestibular impairment and the risk of bilateral vestibulopathy in affected children [29,30]. Future prospective studies and follow-up protocols in children with cCMV should therefore incorporate systematic vestibular assessment alongside audiologic monitoring to provide a more comprehensive evaluation of neurosensory outcomes assessment [31].

This study has several limitations. Its retrospective design and reliance on available medical records may limit generalizability. Only a subset of children diagnosed with cCMV continued audiologic follow-up at our center, introducing selection bias. Children who were more closely monitored or at higher perceived risk were more likely to meet the inclusion criteria, while hearing outcomes for those lost to follow-up or monitored elsewhere were unavailable. Furthermore, the shorter follow-up duration in the normal-hearing group remains a significant limitation, as it may mask the eventual development of late-onset SNHL in some of these children. In addition, incomplete data on maternal serostatus and other perinatal or environmental risk factors limited comprehensive risk stratification. Regarding clinical interventions, the non-randomized allocation of antiviral therapy and variations in treatment duration preclude definitive conclusions regarding its efficacy.

Another limitation relates to the sensitivity of audiologic assessment in early infancy. Children with normal ABR, otoacoustic emissions, and early behavioral thresholds may still have subtle or frequency-specific deficits that are difficult to detect at young ages, raising the possibility of misclassification. Routine sedated ABR for all children with cCMV is neither clinically feasible nor ethically justified, underscoring the inherent challenges of early auditory evaluation in this population.

5. Conclusions

Children with cCMV-related SNHL demonstrate a wide range of hearing trajectories. Hearing loss may present early or late, progress asymmetrically, and evolve differently between ears. The better-ear advantage observed in delayed-onset SNHL, together with the greater tendency toward bilateral and progressive involvement in congenital SNHL, highlights important distinctions between clinical subgroups and reinforces the need for ongoing clinical vigilance throughout childhood. Our findings underscore the necessity of a risk-stratified, long-term surveillance framework that ensures individualized patient monitoring and promotes sustained adherence to follow-up throughout childhood, as missed evaluations may delay recognition of progressive or new hearing loss.

Future prospective studies are needed to establish evidence-based criteria for the duration and intensity of audiologic monitoring across different clinical scenarios, and to clarify how antiviral therapy and early risk markers influence long-term auditory outcomes in children with cCMV.

Author Contributions: Conceptualization, S.S.S., M.K.-Y., R.F., M.G.D. and C.A.; Methodology, S.S.S., M.K.-Y., R.F., M.G.D. and C.A.; Formal analysis, R.F. and M.G.D.; Investigation, R.F. and M.G.D.; Data curation, R.F. and M.G.D.; Writing—original draft preparation, R.F.; Writing—review and editing, M.G.D. and S.S.S.; Visualization, R.F. and S.S.S.; Supervision, S.S.S., M.K.-Y. and C.A. All authors have read and agreed to the published version of the manuscript.

Funding: This research received no external funding.

Institutional Review Board Statement: The study was conducted in accordance with the Declaration of Helsinki and approved by the Institutional Review Board of Hadassah Medical Center (HMO 0495-20; date of approval: 22 June 2020).

Informed Consent Statement: Patient consent was waived due to the retrospective nature of the study and the use of anonymized clinical data.

https://doi.org/10.3390/children13020230

Data Availability Statement: The datasets generated and analyzed during the current study are available from the corresponding author upon reasonable request due to ethical and privacy restrictions.

Acknowledgments: We would like to thank Yarden Zraya and Yarden Levi for their help with data collection.

Conflicts of Interest: The authors declare no conflicts of interest.

Abbreviations

The following abbreviations are used in this manuscript:

ABR	Auditory Brainstem Response
AABR	Automated Auditory Brainstem Response
cCMV	Congenital Cytomegalovirus
CI	Confidence Interval
CPA	Conditioned Play Audiometry
HL	Hearing Loss
HNS	Head and Neck Surgery
IUGR	Intrauterine Growth Restriction
NICU	Neonatal Intensive Care Unit
OR	Odds Ratio
SNHL	Sensorineural Hearing Loss
SRT	Speech Reception Threshold
TEOAEs	Transient-Evoked Otoacoustic Emissions
VRA	Visual Reinforcement Audiometry

References

1. Manicklal, S.; Emery, V.C.; Lazzarotto, T.; Boppana, S.B.; Gupta, R.K. The "silent" global burden of congenital cytomegalovirus. *Clin. Microbiol. Rev.* **2013**, *26*, 86–102. [CrossRef]
2. Schlesinger, Y.; Reich, D.; Eidelman, A.I.; Schimmel, M.S.; Hassanin, J.; Miron, D. Congenital cytomegalovirus infection in Israel: Screening in different subpopulations. *Isr. Med. Assoc. J.* **2005**, *7*, 237–240. [PubMed]
3. Morton, C.C.; Nance, W.E. Newborn Hearing Screening—A Silent Revolution. *N. Engl. J. Med.* **2006**, *354*, 2151–2164. [CrossRef] [PubMed]
4. Goderis, J.; De Leenheer, E.; Smets, K.; Van Hoecke, H.; Keymeulen, A.; Dhooge, I. Hearing loss and congenital CMV infection: A systematic review. *Pediatrics* **2014**, *134*, 972–982. [CrossRef] [PubMed]
5. Lanzieri, T.M.; Chung, W.; Flores, M.; Blum, P.; Caviness, A.C.; Bialek, S.R.; Grosse, S.D.; Miller, J.A.; Demmler-Harrison, G. Hearing Loss in Children With Asymptomatic Congenital Cytomegalovirus Infection. *Pediatrics* **2017**, *139*, e20162610. [CrossRef]
6. Rawlinson, W.D.; Boppana, S.B.; Fowler, K.B.; Kimberlin, D.W.; Lazzarotto, T.; Alain, S.; Daly, K.; Doutré, S.; Gibson, L.; Giles, M.L.; et al. Congenital cytomegalovirus infection in pregnancy and the neonate: Consensus recommendations for prevention, diagnosis, and therapy. *Lancet Infect. Dis.* **2017**, *17*, e177–e188. [CrossRef]
7. Buonsenso, D.; Pedrero-Tomé, R.; Raimondi, F.; Salomé, S.; Papaevangelou, V.; Syridou, G.; Ríos-Barnés, M.; Fortuny, C.; Villaverde, S.; De Vergas, J.; et al. Prognostic Factors of Late-onset Hearing Loss in Infants With Congenital Cytomegalovirus and Normal Audiologic Assessment at Birth. *Pediatr. Infect. Dis. J.* **2025**, *45*, 1–10. [CrossRef]
8. Cheeran, M.C.-J.; Lokensgard, J.R.; Schleiss, M.R. Neuropathogenesis of congenital cytomegalovirus infection: Disease mechanisms and prospects for intervention. *Clin. Microbiol. Rev.* **2009**, *22*, 99–126. [CrossRef]
9. Gabrielli, L.; Bonasoni, M.P.; Piccirilli, G.; Petrisli, E.; Venturoli, S.; Cantiani, A.; Pavoni, M.; Marsico, C.; Capretti, M.G.; Simonazzi, G.; et al. The Auditory Pathway in Congenitally Cytomegalovirus-Infected Human Fetuses. *Int. J. Mol. Sci.* **2024**, *25*, 2636. [CrossRef]
10. Fletcher, K.T.; Horrell, E.M.W.; Ayugi, J.; Irungu, C.; Muthoka, M.; Creel, L.M.; Lester, C.; Bush, M.L. The Natural History and Rehabilitative Outcomes of Hearing Loss in Congenital Cytomegalovirus: A Systematic Review. *Otol. Neurotol.* **2018**, *39*, 854–864. [CrossRef]
11. Xia, W.; Yan, H.; Zhang, Y.; Wang, C.; Gao, W.; Lv, C.; Wang, W.; Liu, Z. Congenital Human Cytomegalovirus Infection Inducing Sensorineural Hearing Loss. *Front. Microbiol.* **2021**, *12*, 649690. [CrossRef] [PubMed]
12. Kenneson, A.; Cannon, M.J. Review and meta-analysis of the epidemiology of congenital cytomegalovirus (CMV) infection. *Rev. Med. Virol.* **2007**, *17*, 253–276. [CrossRef] [PubMed]

https://doi.org/10.3390/children13020230

13. Chatzakis, C.; Ville, Y.; Makrydimas, G.; Dinas, K.; Zavlanos, A.; Sotiriadis, A. Timing of primary maternal cytomegalovirus infection and rates of vertical transmission and fetal consequences. *Am. J. Obstet. Gynecol.* **2020**, *223*, 870–883.e11. [CrossRef] [PubMed]
14. Dollard, S.C.; Grosse, S.D.; Ross, D.S. New estimates of the prevalence of neurological and sensory sequelae and mortality associated with congenital cytomegalovirus infection. *Rev. Med. Virol.* **2007**, *17*, 355–363. [CrossRef]
15. Boppana, S.B.; Ross, S.A.; Fowler, K.B. Congenital cytomegalovirus infection: Clinical outcome. *Clin. Infect. Dis.* **2013**, *57*, S178–S181. [CrossRef]
16. De Cuyper, E.; Acke, F.; Keymeulen, A.; De Leenheer, E.M.R.; Van Hoecke, H.; Padalko, E.; Boudewyns, A.; Gilles, A.; Muylle, M.; Kuhweide, R.; et al. Risk Factors for Hearing Loss at Birth in Newborns With Congenital Cytomegalovirus Infection. *JAMA Otolaryngol. Head. Neck Surg.* **2023**, *149*, 122–130. [CrossRef]
17. Foulon, I.; Vleurinck, L.; Kerkhofs, K.; Gordts, F. Hearing configuration in children with cCMV infection and proposal of a flow chart for hearing evaluation. *Int. J. Audiol.* **2015**, *54*, 714–719. [CrossRef]
18. Royackers, L.; Rector, E.; Verhaert, N.; Desloovere, C. Long-term audiological follow-up of children with congenital cytomegalovirus. *B-ENT* **2013**, *21*, 57–64.
19. Fowler, K.B.; McCollister, F.P.; Sabo, D.L.; Shoup, A.G.; Owen, K.E.; Woodruff, J.L.; Cox, E.; Mohamed, L.S.; Choo, D.I.; Boppana, S.B.; et al. A Targeted Approach for Congenital Cytomegalovirus Screening Within Newborn Hearing Screening. *Pediatrics* **2017**, *139*, e20162128. [CrossRef]
20. Schleiss, M.R. Evolving Concepts in Care for Congenital Cytomegalovirus (cCMV) Infection: Better Outcomes for More Babies! *J. Pediatr.* **2024**, *270*, 114044. [CrossRef]
21. Fowler, K.B.; Boppana, S.B. Congenital cytomegalovirus (CMV) infection and hearing deficit. *J. Clin. Virol.* **2006**, *35*, 226–231. [CrossRef]
22. Goderis, J.; Keymeulen, A.; Smets, K.; Van Hoecke, H.; De Leenheer, E.; Boudewyns, A.; Desloovere, C.; Kuhweide, R.; Muylle, M.; Royackers, L.; et al. Hearing in Children with Congenital Cytomegalovirus Infection: Results of a Longitudinal Study. *J. Pediatr.* **2016**, *172*, 110–115.e2. [CrossRef] [PubMed]
23. Friedman, S.E.; Shlomai, N.O.; Oiknine-Djian, E.; Sido, T.; Gordon, O.; Greenberger, S.; Horowitz, H.; Merav, L.; Mehaber, S.D.; Caplan, O.; et al. Lessons derived from a 3-year congenital cytomegalovirus screening programme in Israel: A prospective population-based cohort study. *Lancet Infect. Dis.* **2025**. Available online: https://cris.huji.ac.il/en/publications/lessons-derived-from-a-3-year-congenital-cytomegalovirus-screenin/ (accessed on 22 December 2025). [CrossRef]
24. Torrecillas, V.; Allen, C.M.; Greene, T.; Park, A.; Chung, W.; Lanzieri, T.M.; Demmler-Harrison, G. Should You Follow the Better-Hearing Ear for Congenital Cytomegalovirus Infection and Isolated Sensorineural Hearing Loss? *Otolaryngol. Head Neck Surg.* **2020**, *162*, 114–120. [CrossRef]
25. Alkoby-Meshulam, L.; Rosenthal-Shtern, D.; Snapiri, O.; Levy, D.; Sachs, N.; Sokolov, M.; Bilavsky, E. Unilateral Sensorineural Hearing Loss in Congenital Cytomegalovirus Retrospective Observational Study. *Pediatr. Infect. Dis. J.* **2025**, *44*, 234–238. [CrossRef] [PubMed]
26. Aldè, M.; Fancello, V.; Mauro, P.D.; Canelli, R.; Zaouche, S.; Falanga, C.; Aldè, M.; Fancello, V.; Mauro, P.D.; Canelli, R.; et al. Audiological and Vestibular Follow-Up for Children with Congenital Cytomegalovirus Infection: From Current Limitations to Future Directions. *Children* **2024**, *11*, 1211. [CrossRef]
27. Korndewal, M.J.; Oudesluys-Murphy, A.M.; Kroes, A.C.M.; van der Sande, M.A.B.; de Melker, H.E.; Vossen, A.C.T.M. Long-term impairment attributable to congenital cytomegalovirus infection: A retrospective cohort study. *Dev. Med. Child. Neurol.* **2017**, *59*, 1261–1268. [CrossRef]
28. Palma, S.; Forli, F.; Rossi, C.; Filice, R.; D'adamo, C.; Roversi, M.F.; Monzani, D.; Lorenzoni, F.; Botti, C.; Berrettini, S.; et al. The Audiological Follow-Up of Children with Symptomatic Congenital Cytomegalovirus Infection: An Experience in Two Italian Centers. *Children* **2023**, *10*, 1136. [CrossRef]
29. Cushing, S.L.; Gordon, K.A.; Rutka, J.A.; James, A.L.; Papsin, B.C. Vestibular end-organ dysfunction in children with sensorineural hearing loss and cochlear implants: An expanded cohort and etiologic assessment. *Otol. Neurotol.* **2013**, *34*, 422–428. [CrossRef]
30. Kaski, D.; Tarnutzer, A.A.; Agrawal, Y.; Carey, J.; Cha, Y.-H.; Eggers, S.D.; Furman, J.; Kim, H.A.; Kim, J.-S.; Lempert, T.; et al. The International Classification of Vestibular Disorders: Achievements, challenges, and future directions. *J. Vestib. Res.* **2025**, *35*, 105–112. [CrossRef]
31. Singh, A.; Raynor, E.M.; Lee, J.W.; Smith, S.L.; Heet, H.; Garrison, D.; Wrigley, J.; Kaylie, D.M.; Riska, K.M. Vestibular Dysfunction and Gross Motor Milestone Acquisition in Children With Hearing Loss: A Systematic Review. *Otolaryngol. Head. Neck Surg.* **2021**, *165*, 493–506. [CrossRef]

https://doi.org/10.3390/children13020230

children

MDPI

Article

Advancing Pediatric Cochlear Implant Care Through a Multidisciplinary Telehealth Model: Insights from Implementation and Family Perspectives

Chrisanda Marie Sanchez [1,2,*], Jennifer Coto [1,2], Jordan Ian McNair [1,2], Domitille Lochet [1], Alexandria Susan Mestres [1], Christina Sarangoulis [1], Meredith A. Holcomb [1] and Ivette Cejas [1,2]

1 Department of Otolaryngology, University of Miami, Miami, FL 33136, USA; meredith.holcomb@med.miami.edu (M.A.H.)
2 Department of Pediatrics, University of Miami, Miami, FL 33136, USA
* Correspondence: cmsanchez@med.miami.edu

Abstract

Background/Objectives: Multidisciplinary care is the gold-standard approach for delivering comprehensive pediatric healthcare. For children undergoing cochlear implant (CI) evaluation, multiple appointments are required to assess candidacy, set realistic expectations, and counsel families on rehabilitation and the psychosocial impact of hearing loss. Established pediatric CI users also need coordinated follow-up to address ongoing auditory, educational, and psychosocial needs. This study evaluated the satisfaction and family perspectives of the implementation of a virtual, team-based multidisciplinary model for both CI candidates and established CI users. Methods: Thirty-nine children and their families participated in discipline-specific telehealth consultations, including audiology, listening and spoken language (LSL) therapy, psychology, and educational services, followed by a 60 min multidisciplinary team meeting. Team meetings occurred during pre-implantation and at six months post-activation for CI candidates. Team meetings for established CI users were scheduled following completion of individual consultations. Providers summarized findings from their individual visits before transitioning to a caregiver-led discussion. Post-visit surveys assessed satisfaction and perceived benefit from the multidisciplinary model. Results: Thirty-nine dyads were enrolled (11 Pre-CI; 28 Established CI). Caregivers were predominantly mothers (89.7%), most identified as Hispanic (55.3%) and White (71.1%). Over half of children identified as Hispanic (59%) and White (71.8%); most were diagnosed with hearing loss at birth (55.9%). Satisfaction with the virtual model was uniformly high: 100% of caregivers were satisfied or very satisfied, and most rated care quality as "very good" or "excellent." LSL therapy was most frequently rated as the most beneficial visit (70% Pre-CI; 45% Established CI). Caregivers strongly preferred ongoing team-based care, with 55–80% reporting that they would like it to occur every six months and 95–100% preferring remote meetings. Conclusions: A virtual multidisciplinary model offers a high-quality, family-centered approach for both CI evaluations and ongoing management of established CI users. By integrating simultaneous team-based sessions, this model not only supports the 'whole child' but also strengthens the family system by improving communication, streamlining care, and reducing the burden of multiple in-person appointments. Families consistently report high levels of satisfaction with the convenience, clarity, and collaboration provided through virtual team visits. Incorporating routine check-ins with families is essential to ensure their needs are addressed, reinforce progress, and guide timely, targeted interventions that maximize each child's developmental outcomes.

Children **2026**, *12*, 39 https://doi.org/10.3390/children12010039

Keywords: cochlear implants; pediatric audiology; telehealth; multidisciplinary care; remote programming

1. Introduction

Children with hearing loss are at increased risk for delays in speech and language development [1–5], psychosocial functioning [6,7], educational outcomes [8–10], and overall quality of life [9,11]. Timely and appropriate intervention is essential to mitigate these risks. The Joint Committee on Infant Hearing (JCIH) recommends the 1-3-6 benchmark where children should be screened by 1 month, diagnosed by 3 months, and enrolled in early intervention by 6 months [12]. Effective care requires multiple appointments from diagnosis through follow-up. Many children with hearing loss also have comorbid medical conditions [13,14], further increasing the number of necessary visits. Innovative care models are needed to improve outcomes while reducing family burden.

The American Academy of Pediatrics identifies team-based care as the gold standard for managing pediatric healthcare [15]. Children with complex or chronic medical conditions often require care that addresses not only their primary diagnosis, but also the broader impact on development, behavior, and family well-being [16–19]. Multidisciplinary care integrates expertise from multiple healthcare professionals to create individualized, comprehensive care plans. Such models have demonstrated success in other pediatric fields, including craniofacial anomalies [20], oncology tumor boards [21], and pediatric oncology [22]. Although the literature in pediatric audiology is more limited, studies report high caregiver satisfaction with traditional in-person multidisciplinary models [23,24].

This study evaluates a telehealth-based model for managing pediatric hearing loss in children pre- or post-cochlear implantation (CI). Traditional CI teams include audiology, speech therapy, and otolaryngology. In our model, the team also includes psychology, listening and spoken language (LSL) therapy, and an educational specialist to provide more comprehensive support.

Telehealth allows families to access healthcare from home via electronic devices (e.g., laptop, cellphone). Interest in telehealth has grown substantially in recent years [25,26], particularly during the COVID-19 pandemic. With the expected increase in hearing loss [27] prevalence, efficient and scalable care models are needed. Prior studies show that telehealth can reduce in-person visits while maintaining outcomes, particularly for remote CI programming and audiology services [26,28,29]. However, these studies primarily focus on audiology and do not include the full multidisciplinary team needed for pediatric hearing loss management.

Despite the growing use of telehealth for audiologic services and remote CI programming, few studies have examined its feasibility or implementation within a truly comprehensive multidisciplinary framework that incorporates audiology, speech-language pathology, psychology, and educational services. These additional disciplines are essential for understanding the broader developmental, behavioral, emotional, and academic needs of children with hearing loss, needs that cannot be fully captured through audiologic testing alone. Psychologists offer expertise in socioemotional functioning and family well-being, while educational specialists evaluate classroom performance, communication access, and early learning skills. Traditionally, accessing this range of expertise requires families to attend multiple in-person appointments across different clinics and service systems, which creates substantial logistical challenges and makes coordination difficult for providers. A virtual delivery model has the potential to reduce these barriers by bringing the full team together in a single, accessible encounter. This approach supports more holistic assessment,

https://doi.org/10.3390/children12010039

more efficient care coordination, and earlier identification of developmental or educational concerns that may influence CI outcomes.

Accordingly, this study aimed to (1) evaluate the implementation of a fully remote, multidisciplinary CI team model for pediatric candidacy evaluations and for established CI recipients, and (2) examine caregiver satisfaction and perceived accessibility of telehealth-delivered multidisciplinary care.

2. Materials and Methods

2.1. Participants

Participants were assigned to one of two groups: children undergoing CI evaluation (Pre-CI group) and established CI recipients (Established CI group). For both groups, children were included if they were ages 6 months to 12 years old, had caregivers who agreed to the virtual visits, had access to a smartphone or computer, and who speak English and/or Spanish. For the Pre-CI group, children were enrolled once CI candidacy was confirmed using evidence-based practice guidelines on CI candidacy criteria. Children in the Established CI group were enrolled once they had at least 6 months of CI use. All families in the clinic who met the inclusion criteria were approached to participate in this study until the target enrollment number was met. Of note, the clinic serves a large tri-county area, including primarily individuals from diverse and minority backgrounds within both urban and suburban parts of the South Florida areas.

Forty-five participants (15 Pre-CI group, 30 Established CI group) were originally enrolled in the study. Four participants were excluded from data analysis in the Pre-CI group as they either did not proceed with CI or did not complete any study related measures. Two participants in the Established CI group were also excluded as they also did not attend the study visits or complete any measures. Thus, the sample being reported includes 39 pediatric CI candidates and established recipients (see Table 1 for participant demographics). This study was approved by the University of Miami IRB (IRB #20210584). Informed consent was obtained from all participants involved in the study.

Table 1. Questions from the Remote Multidisciplinary Satisfaction Visit questionnaire.

1.	Which of your remote visits with the multi-disciplinary team was most beneficial for you? (Choose one)
2.	How satisfied were you with the overall multi-disciplinary team meeting?
3.	How important is it for your child's providers to work together?
4.	How well do you think the entire team was on the same page about your child's care?
5.	Which specialists would you like to see again? (Select all)
6.	How often would you like to meet with the multidisciplinary team?
7.	Would you prefer to meet with the multi-disciplinary team members individually or as a group?
8.	Would you want these visits to be remote or in-person?

2.2. Procedures

Participants were identified and approached by their clinical audiologist to participate in the multidisciplinary telehealth study. All participants completed discipline-specific telehealth consultations, which included audiology, LSL therapy, psychology, and educational services. Each consultation was conducted via a secure telehealth platform (Zoom) and focused on discipline-specific assessment and recommendations (see detailed explanations of each consultation below). Following the individual consultations, a virtual team meeting was scheduled. For established CI recipients, a multidisciplinary team meeting followed the completion of these individual sessions. For the Pre-CI group, team meetings were

https://doi.org/10.3390/children12010039

slated to occur pre-implantation and at 6 months post-activation. This study only reports the initial team meeting, as only 50% of the Pre-CI group attended the 6-month team meeting. All multidisciplinary team meetings were attended by the same core group of specialists, ensuring consistent representation from audiology, speech-language pathology, psychology, and education across all visits.

2.3. Audiology

All patients were initially seen in clinic for audiologic enrollment and baseline assessment. For the Pre-CI group, comprehensive evaluations were conducted, including audiometric testing and candidacy determination consistent with standard clinical protocols.

For the Established CI group, children attended their in-person routine visit and then were enrolled in the remote study. Follow-up audiology appointments were completed remotely and included device impedance measurements, electrically evoked compound action potentials (ECAPs), and assessment of overall audibility. These remote sessions additionally incorporated guided discussions between the audiologist, child, and caregiver to evaluate listening performance, device function, and progress toward auditory goals.

2.4. Listening and Spoken Language Therapy

Families in both the Pre-CI and Established CI groups participated in a remote check-in to discuss their child's speech and language development and current concerns. When further evaluation was indicated, children were scheduled for a comprehensive speech and language assessment either in person or via telehealth using a standard protocol. Assessment sessions followed the same structure and duration as in-person visits—60 min for younger children under 2 years and 120 min for those aged 3 and older. Younger children's evaluations included parent interviews, listening activities, and language observation, while older children's sessions included age-appropriate speech and language assessments. All sessions were conducted by a certified listening and spoken language specialist (LSLS Cert. AVT) using evidence-based auditory-verbal strategies in the child's primary language (English, Spanish, or both). For bilingual assessments, therapists followed tele-practice guidelines from each test publisher to ensure standardized administration. Both English and Spanish assessments were administered by speech-language pathologists with documented Spanish fluency and competency, following test manuals to ensure fidelity and accuracy across languages.

2.5. Education Consultation

Each family participated in a consultation via phone or a virtual platform with a deaf and hard-of-hearing (D/HH) educational specialist as part of the multidisciplinary CI evaluation process. Families were asked to provide relevant educational documentation (e.g., Individualized Education Programs [IEPs], Individualized Family Service Plans [IFSPs], or 504 plans) prior to the meeting. During the consultation, the D/HH specialist reviewed the child's educational history, current placement, and academic progress, with discussions tailored according to whether the child was in the Pre-CI Group or Established CI Group. The D/HH specialist identified areas of educational need, provided counseling regarding school-based support, and reviewed appropriate accommodations and interventions aligned with the child's communication and listening goals.

When children lacked existing educational support, discussions focused on available resources and strategies to initiate services, as well as appropriate educational placements. For those with established plans, the discussion focused on optimizing current support and addressing ongoing challenges. Each session concluded with a summary of recommendations and key points to be communicated to the multidisciplinary CI team.

https://doi.org/10.3390/children12010039

2.6. Psychology Consultation

Psychology consultations were conducted remotely and lasted approximately 30 to 60 min. The primary purpose of these visits was to assess each child's functioning across academic, social, emotional, and behavioral domains. When no current concerns were reported by the family, the consultation served as an opportunity to provide education on the available psychology services and how to access them in the future if needed. When parents or caregivers identified concerns related to their child's behavior, mood, learning, or adjustment, additional information was obtained to clarify the nature and extent of the difficulties. Based on this initial screening, follow-up services were arranged as appropriate, including individual or family therapy, or a comprehensive psychoeducational evaluation to assess potential learning, attention, or neurodevelopmental disorders.

2.7. Multidisciplinary Team Meeting

Multidisciplinary team meetings were held via Zoom for approximately 60 min and included the audiologist, LSLS Cert. AVT speech-language pathologist, psychologist, educational specialist, and parent. During the team visit, findings from each provider were reviewed in the context of the child's broader medical, audiological, developmental, and therapeutic care. Providers briefly summarized findings and recommendations from their individual consultations, after which the discussion shifted to a parent-led discussion to address priorities and concerns. Based on the multidisciplinary discussion, individualized recommendations were formulated, and appropriate referrals for follow-up services were provided as indicated. At the conclusion of the visit, parents were invited to complete a brief survey evaluating their satisfaction with the multidisciplinary telehealth experience, including perceived coordination of care, communication among providers, and the relevance of recommendations to their child's needs (all survey questions and responses can be found in the Supplemental Table S3a–c).

2.8. Virtual Team Visit Satisfaction

Caregivers in both cohorts completed post-visit surveys assessing the acceptability of and satisfaction with the virtual multidisciplinary model. A brief family satisfaction survey was administered through Qualtrics to evaluate caregiver satisfaction of the virtual multidisciplinary team visit. The eight-item survey included a mix of response formats, including multiple-choice questions and Likert-scale ratings (see Table 1). Families accessed and completed the survey directly through the Qualtrics platform, which could be completed on a computer, tablet, or smartphone at their convenience with a unique survey access code. This format allowed flexible participation and ensured that responses were collected in a secure, standardized manner. All questions from the Virtual Team Visit with their results can be found in Supplemental Table S3a–c.

3. Results

3.1. Demographics

A total of 39 parent–child dyads participated in the study (11 Pre-CI and 28 in Established CI). In the Pre-CI group, eleven patients (54.5% female) with a mean age of 4.29 years (SD = 4.15) and their caregivers (all mothers) were enrolled. Caregivers had a mean age of 33.11 years (SD = 5.28); 63.6% were married and most identified as Hispanic (54.5%) and/or White (72.7%). Nearly half (45.5%) reported holding a graduate degree, and 27.3% were working on-site at the time of the study. Among the children, 54.5% identified as Hispanic and 63.6% as White. Over half (54.5%) were diagnosed with hearing loss at birth, all had been fit with hearing aids, and 63.6% received their initial hearing aid fitting after 12 months of age.

https://doi.org/10.3390/children12010039

In the Established CI group, twenty-eight patients (42.9% female) with a mean age of 6.43 years (SD = 3.16) and their caregivers (85.7% mothers) were enrolled. Caregivers had a mean age of 38 years (SD = 9.13), and the majority were married (59.3%). Most caregivers identified as Hispanic (55.6%) and/or White (70.4%). The most reported highest education level was a bachelor's degree (33.3%), and 44.4% were working on-site.

Among the children, 63% identified as Hispanic and 74.1% as White. Most were diagnosed with hearing loss at birth (55.6%), and 88.9% had been fit with hearing aids. Hearing aid fitting typically occurred between 6 and 12 months of age (34.8%) or after 12 months (34.8%). Further demographic information for the Established CI group is presented in Table 2.

Table 2. Sample Characteristics.

	Pre-CI $n = 11$	**Established CI** $n = 28$
Characteristic	**Mean (*SD*)**	**Mean (*SD*)**
Child Age	4.29 (*4.15*)	6.43 (*3.16*)
Caregiver age	33.11 (*5.28*)	38.00 (9.13)
Characteristic	***n* (%)**	***n* (%)**
Caregiver relationship to child		
Mother	11 (100%)	24 (85.7%)
Father	0 (0%)	4 (14.3%)
Caregiver marital status		
Married	7 (63.6%)	16 (59.3%)
Separated	0 (0%)	3 (11.1%)
Living with partner	3 (27.3%)	1 (3.7%)
Single	1 (9.1%)	7 (25.9%)
Caregiver race		
White	8 (72.7%)	19 (70.4%)
Black	3 (27.3%)	5 (18.5%)
Asian	0 (0%)	1 (3.7%)
Other	0 (0%)	2 (7.4%)
Caregiver ethnicity		
Non-Hispanic	5 (45.5%)	12 (44.4%)
Hispanic	6 (54.5%)	15 (55.6%)
Caregiver highest education		
Less than high school	1 (9.1%)	0 (0%)
High school	2 (18.2%)	1 (3.7%)
Technical school	1 (9.1%)	1 (3.7%)
Some college/no degree	0 (0%)	4 (14.8%)
Associate's degree	1 (9.1%)	6 (22.2%)
Bachelor's degree	1 (9.1%)	9 (33.3%)
Graduate degree	5 (45.5%)	6 (22.2%)
Caregiver employment status		
Unemployed	1 (9.1%)	5 (18.5%)
Working from home	2 (18.2%)	4 (14.8%)
Self-employed	1 (9.1%)	0 (0%)
Working on site	3 (27.3%)	12 (44.4%)
Combination: home/on site	2 (18.2%)	3 (11.1%)
Homemaker	2 (18.2%)	3 (11.1%)

https://doi.org/10.3390/children12010039

Table 2. *Cont.*

	Pre-CI *n* = 11	Established CI *n* = 28
Characteristic	**Mean (*SD*)**	**Mean (*SD*)**
Child Age	4.29 (*4.15*)	6.43 (*3.16*)
Caregiver age	33.11 (*5.28*)	38.00 (9.13)
Characteristic	***n* (%)**	***n* (%)**
Child Sex		
Female	6 (54.5%)	12 (42.9%)
Male	5 (45.5%)	16 (57.1%)
Child Race		
White	7 (63.6%)	20 (74.1%)
Black	3 (27.3%)	4 (14.8%)
Asian	0 (0%)	1 (3.7%)
Other	1 (9.1%)	2 (7.4%)
Child Ethnicity		
Non-Hispanic	5 (45.5%)	10 (37.0%)
Hispanic	6 (54.5%)	17 (63.0%)
Child diagnosed with hearing loss		
At birth	6 (54.5%)	15 (55.6%)
Before 3 months	0 (0%)	4 (14.8%)
Between 6 and 12 months	0 (0%)	2 (7.4%)
Other age	5 (45.5%)	6 (22.2%)
CI recommended (age)		
Before 3 months	1 (9.1%)	1 (3.7%)
Between 3 and 6 months	0 (0%)	6 (22.2%)
Between 6 and 12 months	3 (27.3%)	5 (18.5%)
Other age	7 (63.6%)	15 (55.6%)
Child fit with hearing aids		
Yes	11 (100%)	24 (88.9%)
No	0 (0%)	3 (11.1%)
Fit with hearing aids (age)		
Before 3 months	0 (0%)	1 (4.3%)
Between 3 and 6 months	4 (36.4%)	6 (26.1%)
Between 6 and 12 months	0 (0%)	8 (34.8%)
Other age	7 (63.6%)	8 (34.8%)

Full demographic information is presented in Table 2.

3.2. *Survey Results*

A subset of participants missed the team meeting; thus, the survey results reflect the number of those who attended. In the Pre-CI group, four additional enrolled participants (26.6% of the total) were excluded due to incomplete surveys or not proceeding with CI. In the Established CI group, two participants were excluded for missing most appointments, and five of the remaining 28 missed the team meeting (17.8%).

Given the small sample size and limited variability in responses, all survey data are presented using descriptive statistics. Comparative statistical testing (e.g., chi-square, t-test) was not appropriate, as several contingency cells contained very low counts, which could violate assumptions and produce unstable estimates. Descriptive measures, including frequencies, percentages, means, and standard deviations, provide an accurate summary of caregiver responses and observed trends across the Pre-CI and Established CI groups. All questions and results can be found in Supplemental Tables S1–S3.

https://doi.org/10.3390/children12010039

3.3. Technology Use

In the Pre-CI group, most caregivers reported using the following on a daily basis: a smartphone (100%) or computer/tablet (90%); checking email (100%), sending emails (70%), and sending text messages (90%). Half of caregivers reported regularly using a video conferencing service (50%) or using Bluetooth technology to pair their devices (80%). Four caregivers disagreed that people close to them would refer to them as "tech savvy" (40%) and one caregiver agreed that they are easily frustrated by technology (10%).

Similarly, in the Established CI group, most caregivers reported daily smartphone use (91.3%) and more than half used a computer or tablet each day (65.2%). Regular communication tasks were also common, including checking email (91.3%), sending emails (65.2%), and texting (87%). Many caregivers routinely used video-conferencing platforms (69.6%) and paired devices via Bluetooth (78.2%). Despite this frequent technology use, 43.5% of caregivers disagreed that people close to them would describe them as "tech savvy," and one caregiver (4.3%) strongly agreed that they are easily frustrated by technology.

Overall, both groups demonstrated sufficient technology skills to participate effectively in virtual multidisciplinary visits. All participants scheduled for the virtual team meeting were able to access the session without technical issues. All technology questions and results are highlighted in Supplemental Table S1.

3.4. Visit Time Burden

Caregivers in both groups generally reported that attending appointments was manageable, though ease differed between groups. In the Pre-CI group, most caregivers agreed or strongly agreed that it was easy to attend their appointment (81.8%) and to arrive on time (63.6%). In contrast, just over half of caregivers in the Established CI group agreed or strongly agreed that attending their appointment (51.9%) and arriving on time (51.9%) was easy.

Time off from work also varied by group. In the Pre-CI group, half of caregivers reported taking some time off work, with 54.5% reporting no time off, 9.1% taking 2–4 h, 18.2% taking 4–6 h, and 18.2% taking 6–8 h; 60% of caregivers used unpaid time off. Among the Established CI group, most caregivers did not take time off (85.7%), while 10.7% took 4–6 h and 3.6% took 6–8 h; 75% of caregivers used paid time off.

Regarding patients, three in the Pre-CI group (27.3%) and five in the Established CI group (17.9%) had to take time off school to attend the appointment. Additionally, half of Pre-CI caregivers (50%) and 14.3% of Established CI caregivers had to coordinate with someone else to watch other children or dependents. All Visit Time Burden questions and their results are highlighted in Supplemental Table S2a.

3.5. Caregiver Satisfaction

Caregiver satisfaction with the clinic visit was high in both groups. All caregivers in both the Pre-CI and Established CI groups reported being "satisfied" or "very satisfied" with their visit. Most caregivers in the Pre-CI group rated the quality of care as "very good" or "excellent" (90.9%), while all caregivers in the Established CI group rated the quality of care as "very good" or "excellent" (100%). Similarly, the majority of caregivers reported that their provider spent "just the right" amount of time with them: 90.9% in the Pre-CI group and 96.3% in the Established CI group. All Caregiver Satisfaction questions and their results are highlighted in Supplemental Table S2b.

3.6. Multidisciplinary Team Meeting

For multidisciplinary team meetings, caregivers in both groups endorsed high satisfaction and perceived importance of collaboration. In the Pre-CI group, all caregivers were "extremely satisfied" (100%) and endorsed that it was "extremely" important for all their child's providers to work together. Speech therapy was identified as the most beneficial visit (70%), followed by psychology (20%) and educational specialist (10%). Most caregivers wanted to see all specialists again, including the speech therapist (90%), psychologist (70%), and educational specialist (70%; See Figure 1). Caregivers preferred follow-up every six months, representing 80% of the group, favored remote meetings, representing 100%, and preferred team-based meetings at 90% rather than individual specialist visits.

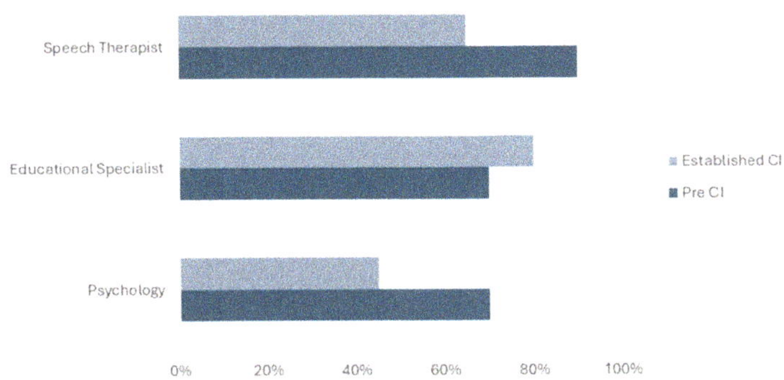

Figure 1. Which specialists would you like to see again?

In the Established CI group, 95% of caregivers were "extremely satisfied" with the multidisciplinary team meeting and 5% were "somewhat satisfied." All caregivers endorsed that provider collaboration was "extremely" important. Speech therapy was identified as the most beneficial (45%), followed by educational specialist (35%) and psychology (20%; See Figure 1). Caregivers wanted to see all specialists again, including the educational specialist (80%), speech therapist (65%), and psychologist (45%). Caregivers preferred follow-up every six months, representing 55% of the group, favored remote meetings at 95% and half preferred team-based meetings while the other half were equally willing to meet with individual specialists.

Comparative observations between the groups revealed that Pre-CI caregivers placed greater emphasis on LSL therapy as the most beneficial (70% vs. 45% in Established CI) and were more likely to prefer seeing all specialists again. In contrast, caregivers in the Established CI group placed relatively greater emphasis on the educational specialist visits (35% vs. 10%). Follow-up preferences also differed: Pre-CI caregivers more frequently preferred six-month intervals (80% vs. 55%) and team-based meetings (90% vs. 50%), whereas half of the Established CI cohort were equally willing to meet with individual specialists. Despite these differences, satisfaction ratings and the perceived importance of provider collaboration remained consistently high across both groups. All Multidisciplinary Team Visit satisfaction and preference questions and their results are highlighted in Supplemental Table S3a–c.

Overall, virtual multidisciplinary CI care was associated with high caregiver satisfaction, adequate technology use, and manageable logistical burden. Patterns differed across Pre-CI and Established CI groups, highlighting the importance of stage-specific, tailored multidisciplinary support.

Figure 1 highlights which specialists each group preferred seeing again following their virtual visit excluding audiology (as this is considered a required specialty for pediatric CI care).

https://doi.org/10.3390/children12010039

4. Discussion

This study evaluated the implementation of a virtual multidisciplinary model for pediatric CI evaluation and follow-up care. We also assessed caregiver satisfaction and accessibility of telehealth services. Our findings show that this approach can effectively integrate multiple disciplines into a coordinated virtual format, maintaining quality of care while enhancing family engagement.

Nearly all caregivers reported being "very satisfied" with the team-based telehealth format and rated the quality of care as "excellent." High satisfaction with virtual delivery and desire for regular team meetings highlight the value of this model in improving accessibility and reducing the logistical burden of care. These results support telehealth as a promising strategy to address access disparities and improve efficiency in pediatric CI care.

Traditional multidisciplinary CI care typically requires multiple in-person appointments over several days or weeks [30]. While effective, these models can create challenges for families, including travel time, missed work, and coordination with school schedules [31,32]. The virtual model consolidates multiple provider perspectives into a single meeting, reducing the in-person visits without sacrificing quality of care. This aligns with previous research showing that remote CI programming can achieve high patient satisfaction and outcomes comparable to in-person services [26].

Telehealth offers unique advantages for pediatric CI programs. It reduces travel burden, increases access for families living far from implant centers, and allows for the inclusion of caregivers or educational team members who may not regularly attend in-person appointments [26,29]. This model also promotes real-time interdisciplinary communication, ensuring consistency in recommendations and care plans [33]. Strong parental satisfaction for remote delivery suggests that virtual models may support long-term engagement with the CI team, potentially improving adherence to rehabilitation plans and follow-up schedules.

This study also highlights the value of proactive multidisciplinary care. Families can access specialized expertise before concerns become critical. Traditionally, specialties such as psychology and education are engaged only when problems arise. In this model, remote team meetings allowed early identification and discussion of developmental, behavioral, or educational needs. Families reported high satisfaction with this proactive approach, with most expressing interest in ongoing follow-up sessions, reflecting that they viewed coordinated multidisciplinary input as a useful component of their child's ongoing care, even if no specific concerns were present at the time. Subgroup differences further emphasize the importance of individualized care. Families of children in the Established CI group often identified the educational component as the most beneficial and wanted continued follow-up. Contrarily, families in the Pre-CI group most frequently valued LSL services. These differences reflect developmental stages of children and clinical priorities: children with established CI focus on educational performance, while those undergoing CI evaluation are developing auditory and spoken language skills. These findings reinforce the need to tailor multidisciplinary discussions to each child's developmental level and stage in the intervention process.

Families also rated the final team meeting positively. Survey items specifically asked caregivers how well the multidisciplinary team appeared "on the same page" and how important it was for their child's providers to work together. Caregivers reported that hearing a unified message from multiple specialists clarified next steps, minimized confusion, and strengthened confidence in the care plan. This collaborative wrap-up appears to be a key feature of the model, enhancing family understanding, satisfaction, and perceived continuity of care. These findings align with research conducted by Albertson and colleagues [34]

https://doi.org/10.3390/children12010039

demonstrating that clear and coordinated messages from the care team enhance caregivers' understanding and overall satisfaction.

5. Limitations

Despite these advantages, several challenges remain. While our findings suggest that virtual multidisciplinary CI care is feasible and well-received, the study's single-center design and relatively small sample limit generalizability. Further research across multiple sites with larger samples is needed to confirm these results and support broader implementation. Telehealth delivery depends on reliable internet, access to devices, and caregiver familiarity with virtual platforms. While most participants reported regular technology use, the cohort may underrepresent families with limited access, lower digital literacy, or constrained socioeconomic resources, who may face additional barriers to participating fully in virtual care. Addressing these digital and socioeconomic factors is critical to ensuring equitable access, and future studies should explore strategies such as device or internet provision, caregiver training in telehealth platforms, and flexible scheduling to support diverse populations. Some assessments, particularly in speech and language, required modifications for remote administration, and not all tools are formally validated for telemedicine. Certain audiologic care tasks, such as device troubleshooting or programming adjustments, still require in-person visits.

Billing and reimbursement also present important considerations for broader implementation. Because this project was conducted as a research study, the virtual multidisciplinary visits were not billed to insurance, and no clinical billing codes were applied. In standard clinical settings, however, reimbursement remains a significant barrier. Existing payer structures often do not support integrated, multi-provider telehealth encounters. For example, commonly used telehealth evaluation and management codes, time-based behavioral health codes, and therapy service codes are typically structured for single-provider visits and may not allow simultaneous or sequential same-day billing across multiple disciplines. Some insurers also restrict reimbursement for extended multidisciplinary case discussions or require in-person components for coverage. These limitations may constrain scalability in routine care. Establishing feasible billing pathways and evaluating the cost-effectiveness of multidisciplinary telehealth models will be essential for sustainable implementation beyond the research context.

Finally, a subset of participants (15.6%) missed several appointments, including the final team meeting. Reasons for missed visits were unknown, highlighting ongoing challenges in coordinating multidisciplinary care. Despite these limitations, structured proactive check-ins provide meaningful benefits for families who seek to engage with the full team.

Future Directions

Our results support broader adoption of virtual multidisciplinary care for pediatric CI programs. Future work should validate remote assessment protocols, expand access to remote programming technologies, and explore reimbursement models to support sustainability. Multi-center trials could evaluate scalability and outcomes across populations and health systems. Integrating virtual multidisciplinary care into standard practice has the potential to improve access, enhance family-centered care, and optimize long-term outcomes. This project underscores the value of a comprehensive multidisciplinary team, including audiology, LSL therapy, psychology, and education. Structured "check-in" visits allow teams to identify needs proactively. In many cases, children categorized as "good performers" did not report any notable concerns; yet challenges emerged and became apparent when directly assessed by the team or through surveys and discussion. Routine

https://doi.org/10.3390/children12010039

check-ins, whether virtual or in person, help uncover unmet needs, align recommendations, and prompt timely referrals.

Overall, virtual multidisciplinary CI care improves access, achieves high family satisfaction, and identifies needs that vary across the implant journey. Differences between evaluation and post-implant groups highlight the importance of adaptable, stage-specific care models. Addressing ongoing barriers such as reimbursement and telehealth validation will be essential for wider adoption. These findings support a scalable, sustainable, and family-centered framework for virtual multidisciplinary CI management.

6. Conclusions

A virtual multidisciplinary CI care model unites core pediatric hearing healthcare specialists in a single coordinated session, reducing travel and scheduling burdens while enhancing team communication. Families report high satisfaction with this collaborative, streamlined approach, which enables earlier identification of needs and clearer guidance throughout the CI journey. Together these strengths highlight virtual multidisciplinary care as a scalable, equitable, and family-centered strategy for delivering high-quality CI services.

Supplementary Materials: The following supporting information can be downloaded at: https://www.mdpi.com/article/10.3390/children12010039/s1. Table S1: Caregiver Technology Use and Comfort Questions and Results. Table S2a: Time, Work, School, and Care Coordination Burden Questions and Results. Table S2b: Caregiver Satisfaction with In-Person Clinic Visit Questions and Results. Table S3a: Multidisciplinary Team Satisfaction Questions and Results. Table S3b: Caregiver Preferences for Multidisciplinary Team Questions and Results. Tables S3c: Caregiver Preferences for Multidisciplinary Team Follow-Up Questions and Results.

Author Contributions: Conceptualization, C.M.S., I.C., M.A.H., J.C.; Methodology, C.M.S., I.C., M.A.H., J.C.; Validation, C.M.S., I.C., J.C., C.S.; Formal Analysis, J.C., I.C., C.M.S.; Investigation, C.M.S., J.I.M., D.L., A.S.M., J.C., M.A.H., I.C., C.S.; Resources, C.S.; Data Curation, C.M.S., C.S., J.C.; Writing—Original Draft Preparation, C.M.S., J.I.M., J.C., D.L., A.S.M.; Writing—Review and Editing, M.A.H., I.C.; Visualization, C.M.S., I.C.; Supervision, C.M.S., I.C.; Project Administration, C.S.; Funding Acquisition, C.M.S. All authors have read and agreed to the published version of the manuscript.

Funding: This research was funded by University of Miami Stanley J. Glaser Grant; Award number UM SJG 2022-15.

Institutional Review Board Statement: The study was conducted in accordance with the Declaration of Helsinki and approved by the Institutional Review Board of University of Miami protocol code 20210584; approved on 8 December 2021.

Informed Consent Statement: Informed consent was obtained from all subjects involved in the study.

Data Availability Statement: The original contributions presented in this study are included in the article/Supplementary Materials. Further inquiries can be directed to the corresponding author.

Conflicts of Interest: C.M.S.—Cochlear research grant; J.C.—MED-EL research grant; J.I.M—Consultant for MED-EL and Institute for Cochlear Implant Training; D.L.—none; A.S.M.—none; C.M.S.—none; M.A.H.—Cochlear and MED-EL research grants, consultant for Advanced Bionics, Cochlear, MED-EL, Hemideina, Institute for Cochlear Implant Training, and Akouos; I.C.—Cochlear, Regeneron, NIH research grants, consultant for Regeneron and Cochlear; The conflicts of interest had no role in the design of the study; in the collection, analyses, or interpretation of data; in the writing of the manuscript; or in the decision to publish the results.

References

1. Geers, A.E.; Nicholas, J.G. Enduring advantages of early cochlear implantation for spoken language development. *J. Speech Lang. Hear. Res.* **2013**, *56*, 643–655. [CrossRef]

https://doi.org/10.3390/children12010039

2. Dettman, S.J.; Dowell, R.C.; Choo, D.; Arnott, W.; Abrahams, Y.; Davis, A.; Dornan, D.; Leigh, J.; Constantinescu, G.; Cowan, R.; et al. Long-term communication outcomes for children receiving cochlear implants younger than 12 months. *Otol. Neurotol.* **2016**, *37*, e82–e95. [CrossRef]
3. Stika, C.J.; Eisenberg, L.S.; Carter, A.S.; Johnson, K.C.; Ganguly, D.M.H.; Henning, S.C.; DesJardin, J.L. Developmental outcomes in Early-Identified children who are hard of hearing at 2 to 3 years of age. *Ear Hear.* **2021**, *42*, 1238–1252. [CrossRef]
4. Markman, T.M.; Quittner, A.L.; Eisenberg, L.S.; Tobey, E.A.; Thal, D.; Niparko, J.K.; Wang, N. Language development after cochlear implantation: An epigenetic model. *J. Neurodev. Disord.* **2011**, *3*, 388–404. [CrossRef]
5. Ching, T.Y.C.; Dillon, H. Major findings of the LOCHI study on children at 3 years of age and implications for audiological management. *Int. J. Audiol.* **2013**, *52* (Suppl. S2), S65–S68. [CrossRef]
6. Wong, C.L.; Ching, T.Y.C.; Cupples, L.; Button, L.; Leigh, G.; Marnane, V.; Whitfield, J.; Gunnourie, M.; Martin, L. Psychosocial development in 5-Year-Old children with hearing loss using hearing aids or cochlear implants. *Trends Hear.* **2017**, *21*, 2331216517710373. [CrossRef] [PubMed]
7. Polat, F. Factors affecting psychosocial adjustment of deaf students. *J. Deaf Stud. Deaf Educ.* **2003**, *8*, 325–339. [CrossRef]
8. Teasdale, T.W.; Sorensen, M.H. Hearing loss in relation to educational attainment and cognitive abilities: A population study. *Int. J. Audiol.* **2007**, *46*, 172–175. [CrossRef] [PubMed]
9. Cejas, I.; Barker, D.H.; Petruzzello, E.; Sarangoulis, C.M.; Quittner, A.L. Cochlear implantation and Educational and Quality-of-Life Outcomes in Adolescence. *JAMA Otolaryngol.–Head Neck Surg.* **2023**, *149*, 708–715. [CrossRef] [PubMed]
10. Idstad, M.; Engdahl, B. Childhood Sensorineural hearing loss and Educational Attainment in Adulthood: Results from the HUNT study. *Ear Hear.* **2019**, *40*, 1359–1367. [CrossRef]
11. Haukedal, C.L.; Lyxell, B.; Wie, O.B. Health-Related Quality of Life with Cochlear Implants: The Children's Perspective. *Ear Hear.* **2019**, *41*, 330–343. [CrossRef] [PubMed]
12. American Academy of Pediatrics, Joint Committee of Infant Hearing. Year 2019 position statement: Principles and guidelines for early hearing detection and intervention programs. *J. Early Hear. Detect. Interv.* **2020**, *4*, 1–44. [CrossRef]
13. Olivier, N.; Shepherd, D.A.; Smith, L.; Carew, P.; Paxton, G.A.; Downie, L.; Rose, E.; Dawes, K.; Sung, V. Etiology, comorbidities, and health service use in a clinical cohort of children with hearing loss. *Ear Hear.* **2022**, *43*, 1836–1844. [CrossRef]
14. Wainwright, E.; Pham, H.; Clack, R.; Irvine, N.; Tran, T.T.; Maywood, E.; Rodrigues, S.; Hird, K.; Kuthubutheen, J. Detailed prevalence analysis of medical co-morbidities in paediatric cochlear implant recipients. *Int. J. Pediatr. Otorhinolaryngol.* **2025**, *195*, 112410. [CrossRef] [PubMed]
15. Katkin, J.P.; Kressly, S.J.; Edwards, A.R.; Perrin, J.M.; Kraft, C.A.; Richerson, J.E.; Tieder, J.S.; Wall, L.; Alexander, J.J.; Flanagan, P.J.; et al. Guiding Principles for Team-Based Pediatric care. *Pediatrics* **2017**, *140*, e20171489. [CrossRef]
16. Leach, K.F.; Stack, N.J.; Jones, S. Optimizing the multidisciplinary team to enhance care coordination across the continuum for children with medical complexity. *Curr. Probl. Pediatr. Adolesc. Health Care* **2021**, *51*, 101128. [CrossRef] [PubMed]
17. Children and Youth with Special Health Care Needs (CYSHCN) | MCHB. Available online: https://mchb.hrsa.gov/programs-impact/focus-areas/children-youth-special-health-care-needs-cyshcn (accessed on 1 March 2025).
18. Zonta, J.B.; Okido, A.C.C.; De Lima, B.J.; Martins, B.A.; Looman, W.S.; Lopes-Júnior, L.C.; Silva-Rodrigues, F.M.; De Lima, R.a.G. Stress in Family Caregivers of Children with Chronic Health Conditions: A Case–Control Study. *Children* **2024**, *11*, 1347. [CrossRef]
19. Cohn, L.N.; Pechlivanoglou, P.; Lee, Y.; Mahant, S.; Orkin, J.; Marson, A.; Cohen, E. Health Outcomes of Parents of Children with Chronic Illness: A Systematic Review and Meta-Analysis. *J. Pediatr.* **2020**, *218*, 166–177.e2. [CrossRef]
20. Robin, N.H.; Baty, H.; Franklin, J.; Guyton, F.C.; Mann, J.; Woolley, A.L.; Waite, P.D.; Grant, J. The multidisciplinary evaluation and management of cleft lip and palate. *South. Med. J.* **2006**, *99*, 1111–1120. [CrossRef]
21. Wheless, S.A.; McKinney, K.A.; Zanation, A.M. A prospective study of the clinical impact of a multidisciplinary head and neck tumor board. *Otolaryngol.-Neck Surg.* **2010**, *143*, 650–654. [CrossRef]
22. Cantrell, M.A.; RubleRN, C.K. Multidisciplinary care in pediatric oncology. *J. Multidiscip. Healthc.* **2011**, *4*, 171–181. [CrossRef]
23. Findlen, U.M.; Malhotra, P.S.; Adunka, O.F. Parent Perspectives on Multidisciplinary Pediatric Hearing Healthcare. *Int. J. Pediatr. Otorhinolaryngol.* **2018**, *116*, 141–146. [CrossRef]
24. Hawley, K.A.; Goldberg, D.M.; Anne, S. Utility of a Multidisciplinary Approach to Pediatric Hearing Loss. *Am. J. Otolaryngol.* **2017**, *38*, 547–550. [CrossRef]
25. Evans, T.; Nejman, T.; Stewart, E.; Windmill, I. Increasing pediatric audiology services via Telehealth. *Semin. Hear.* **2021**, *42*, 136–151. [CrossRef]
26. Holcomb, M.A.; Coto, J.; Stern, T.; Sarangoulis, C.M.; Cejas, I.; Sanchez, C.M. Remote care: The future of cochlear implants. *Otol. Neurotol.* **2025**, *46*, 372–380. [CrossRef]
27. World Health Organization: WHO. Deafness and Hearing Loss. Available online: https://www.who.int/news-room/fact-sheets/detail/deafness-and-hearing-loss (accessed on 26 February 2025).

https://doi.org/10.3390/children12010039

28. Holcomb, M.A.; Smeal, M.R. How to teach an "Old dog" new tricks: Improving Clinical Efficiency in a Well-Established Cochlear Implant Program. *Otol. Neurotol.* **2024**, *45*, e735–e742. [CrossRef] [PubMed]
29. Slager, H.K.; Jensen, J.; Kozlowski, K.; Teagle, H.; Park, L.R.; Biever, A.; Mears, M. Remote programming of cochlear implants. *Otol. Neurotol.* **2019**, *40*, e260–e266. [CrossRef]
30. Steps to a Cochlear Implant | American Cochlear Implant Alliance. (n.d.). Available online: https://www.acialliance.org/general/custom.asp?page=StepstoaCochlearImplant (accessed on 1 November 2025).
31. Nassiri, A.M.; Marinelli, J.P.; Sorkin, D.L.; Carlson, M.L. Barriers to adult cochlear implant care in the United States: An analysis of health care delivery. *Semin. Hear.* **2021**, *42*, 311–320. [CrossRef] [PubMed]
32. Drake, M.; Friedland, D.R.; Hamad, B.; Marfowaa, G.; Adams, J.A.; Luo, J.; Flanary, V. Factors associated with delayed referral and hearing rehabilitation for congenital sensorineural hearing loss. *Int. J. Pediatr. Otorhinolaryngol.* **2023**, *175*, 111770. [CrossRef] [PubMed]
33. Nassiri, A.M.; Saoji, A.A.; DeJong, M.D.; Tombers, N.M.; Driscoll, C.L.W.; Neff, B.A.; Haynes, D.S.; Carlson, M.L. Implementation Strategy for Highly-Coordinated Cochlear Implant Care with Remote Programming: The Complete Cochlear Implant Care Model. *Otol. Neurotol.* **2022**, *43*, e916–e923. [CrossRef]
34. Albertson, E.M.; Chuang, E.; O'MAsta, B.; Miake-Lye, I.; Haley, L.A.; Pourat, N. Systematic Review of Care Coordination Interventions Linking Health and Social Services for High-Utilizing Patient Populations. *Popul. Health Manag.* **2021**, *25*, 73–85. [CrossRef] [PubMed]

https://doi.org/10.3390/children12010039

children

MDPI

Article

Implementation and Evaluation of a Newborn Hearing Screening Database in a Resource-Limited Setting: Advantages and Limitations

Krittipong Parangrit [1,2], Jutatip Sillabutra [3], Suwicha Kaewsiri Isaradisaikul [4,*] and Kanokwan Kulprachakarn [1,*]

1 School of Health Sciences Research, Research Institute for Health Sciences, Chiang Mai University, Chiang Mai 50200, Thailand; krittipong_p@cmu.ac.th
2 Otolaryngology Unit, Chiangrai Prachanukroh Hospital, Chiang Rai 57000, Thailand
3 Department of Biostatistics, Faculty of Public Health, Mahidol University, Bangkok 10400, Thailand; jutatip.sil@mahidol.ac.th
4 Department of Otolaryngology, Faculty of Medicine, Chiang Mai University, Chiang Mai 50200, Thailand
* Correspondence: suwicha.kaewsiri@cmu.ac.th (S.K.I.); kanokwan.kul@cmu.ac.th (K.K.)

Highlights

What are the main findings?

- Newborn hearing screening database improved coverage, referrals, and ABR timeliness.
- Enhanced workflow efficiency but limited by data completeness and connectivity with other health information systems.

What are the implications of the main findings?

- Digital database integration strengthens early hearing detection in low-resource set-tings.
- Interoperability and staff training are key for sustainable implementation.

Abstract

Background: Congenital hearing loss affects 1–3 per 1000 newborns and requires early detection to prevent developmental delays. Although Thailand implements universal screening, fragmented data systems limit effectiveness. To address this, Chiangrai Prachanukroh Hospital introduced a dedicated newborn hearing screening (NHS) database in 2023 to improve tracking, coordination, and monitoring in a resource-limited setting. **Objectives:** To evaluate the advantages and limitations of NHS database integration on screening coverage, referral rates, follow-up completion, and diagnostic timeliness. **Methods:** A retrospective analytic study was conducted over 24 months, comparing outcomes before (July 2022–June 2023) and after (July 2023–June 2024) database implementation. Key indicators included screening coverage, follow-up attendance, diagnostic ABR completion, and workflow efficiency, with the study period also encompassing the implementation of the database and adaptations to the screening algorithm. Data were analyzed using the chi-square test and fisher's exact tests, supplemented by qualitative observations of system performance. **Results:** Among 8290 newborns, screening coverage before one month increased from 83.47% to 96.64% ($p < 0.001$), while referral rates decreased from 18.44% to 6.47% ($p < 0.001$). Diagnostic ABR completion improved from 7.41% to 52.63% within three months ($p < 0.001$) and from 59.26% to 84.21% within six months ($p = 0.06$). The database improved workflow coordination, but challenges persisted, including incomplete data, limited interoperability, caregiver-related follow-up barriers, and low hearing-aid uptake. **Conclusions:** Integration of the NHS database, as well as protocol changes, improved screening coverage, referral accuracy, and diagnostic timeliness, but follow-up and early intervention barriers persisted. Continued progress will require stronger interoperability, improved family engagement, and digital infrastructure investment, with tele-audiology and decision-support tools helping expand access and efficiency.

Keywords: database integration; digital health system; newborn hearing screening; resource-limited settings

1. Introduction

Congenital hearing loss, one of the most common sensory disorders in newborns, has an estimated global incidence of 1–3 per 1000 live births, with Thailand reporting a similar prevalence of approximately 1.7 per 1000 live births [1,2]. The consequences of undiagnosed or delayed identification of hearing loss in newborns are profound and enduring. Children with unrecognized hearing impairment are at heightened risk for delayed speech and language development, impaired cognitive skills, reduced academic achievement, and long-term social and emotional difficulties [3,4]. These outcomes are often preventable if hearing loss is detected and managed early in life. In response, many countries have adopted the Early Hearing Detection and Intervention (EHDI) framework, a structured public health approach designed to identify and manage congenital hearing loss during the first months of life. Over the past decade, several low- and middle-income countries (LMICs), including Thailand, have made substantial strides in expanding Universal Newborn Hearing Screening (UNHS) programs. Thailand has implemented a national UNHS program since 2021; however, national performance indicators remain variable across regions. National reports indicate that screening coverage typically ranges from 93.10% to 99.78%, with referral rates between 2.51% and 14.49%, and diagnostic completion within three months ranges from 20.13 to 90.91%, particularly in public hospitals with limited audiology resources [5–7]. Hearing-aid fitting before six months of age is similarly uncommon, reflecting systemic barriers to early intervention. These efforts have been supported by national policies and structured pilot programs under the Ministry of Public Health, which have promoted NHS implementation and digital reporting systems across multiple provinces [8,9]. However, the implementation of UNHS in LMIC settings continues to face critical systemic and operational challenges. Additionally, Thailand's national NHS algorithm underwent a major revision in July 2023, changing from screening within seven days and rescreening at three months to screening within 24–48 h after birth and rescreening at one month. A major barrier lies in the limitations of data collection, tracking, and coordination mechanisms within healthcare institutions. In many resource-limited settings, including tertiary hospitals in Thailand, the absence of integrated digital systems has led to fragmented workflows for hearing screening programs. Prior to the introduction of a dedicated digital platform, Chiangrai Prachanukroh Hospital, a regional tertiary referral center in northern Thailand, relied on google forms and multiple manual spreadsheets, which were used across different units and screening periods to manage data. While accessible, these tools were not designed for longitudinal tracking or interdepartmental coordination. Screening results were often recorded in isolation and required extensive cross-checking for follow-up scheduling. Fragmented data across maternity, pediatric, and audiology services created delays and discrepancies in identifying newborns requiring rescreening or diagnostic ABR testing. The inability to generate automated alerts or unified follow-up lists increased the risk of missed cases. Moreover, the manual nature of reporting limited the hospital's ability to monitor indicators such as screening coverage, referral rates, follow-up return rates, and age at diagnosis. To address these gaps, the

https://doi.org/10.3390/children13010022

hospital implemented a dedicated Newborn Hearing Screening (NHS) database in 2023. This standalone platform centralized data, supported structured entry, and generated follow-up lists, enabling semi-automated workflows and improved tracking. The transition represented a critical turning point, but the actual impact of database implementation on program performance remains insufficiently documented in LMICs. This study evaluated the advantages and limitations of NHS database adoption, focusing on coverage, referral, follow-up tracking, and diagnostic completion, while describing operational improvements and persisting challenges.

2. Materials and Methods

2.1. Study Design

A retrospective analytic study was conducted using 24 months of NHS data at Chiangrai Prachanukroh Hospital. Data were reviewed in two phases: before database integration (July 2022–June 2023) and after database integration (July 2023–June 2024). Newborns who died or were transferred before 1 month of age were excluded from both groups.

2.2. Screening Workflow and Database Integration

Before the introduction of the dedicated NHS database, the NHS workflow followed the 'old' system, which relied on google forms and multiple manual spreadsheets for data entry and tracking. During this pre-integration phase, staff entered demographic information, dates and locations of screening, laterality of testing, TEOAE results (pass/refer) (Sentiero device, Path medical, Germany), and basic risk-factor classification into google forms, which were subsequently exported into Microsoft Excel spreadsheets used as the primary data repository. The screening protocol followed a two-stage TEOAE process prior to audiology referral. Newborns received the first TEOAE screening before hospital discharge, performed by ward nurses. Newborns who passed were discharged from further screening. Those who referred on the first test underwent a second in-hospital TEOAE screening. Newborns who failed both screenings were scheduled for outpatient TEOAE rescreening at the Otolaryngology unit, where an audiologist conducted the assessment. Newborns who passed the outpatient rescreening were discharged, whereas those who continued to fail were referred for diagnostic evaluation, including auditory brainstem response (ABR) testing (SmartEP device, Intelligent Hearing Systems, Miami, FL, USA). The audiology team manually cross-checked records against paper files, prepared follow-up lists for rescreening or diagnostic ABR, and scheduled appointments by phone or handwritten notes.

In the post-integration phase, the program was purpose-built for NHS and developed through a national research initiative in Thailand, later adopted at Chiangrai Prachanukroh Hospital. The NHS database is a web-based platform integrated into the hospital intranet. Screening nurses enter OAE results at the point of care using structured data fields, including demographic information, screening result status, and next appointment dates, while automated completeness checks flag missing or inconsistent entries. For newborns requiring rescreening, the system automatically generates daily and weekly follow-up lists and alerts staff when repeat testing is due. Audiologists record diagnostic ABR results directly into the system, allowing real-time status updates. Automated functions include generation of follow-up lists, overdue alerts, and pre-allocated ABR appointment queues, although verification of caregiver attendance remains semi-manual. The platform demonstrated minimal downtime, and staff were trained through a brief one-hour session with supervised practice, allowing structured and reliable data capture to support program evaluation.

https://doi.org/10.3390/children13010022

2.3. Statistical Analysis

Categorical differences between the two groups were analyzed in SPSS version 21, with statistical significance set at $p < 0.05$. Screening coverage, referral rates, and follow-up completion were evaluated using chi-square analysis, while diagnostic outcomes were assessed with Fisher's exact procedure because of small cell sizes.

3. Results

As shown in Figure 1, during the pre-database integration period, 4090 newborns were delivered, of whom 3414 (83.47%) underwent hearing screening before 1 month of age. Of these, 2799 (81.56%) newborns passed the initial TEOAE screening and 633 (18.44%) were referred. Among those referred, 278 (44.99%) newborns were lost to follow-up, while 355 (56.08%) attended rescreening, resulting in 54 newborns (66.67%) completing diagnostic ABR. Only 4 (7.41%) newborns achieved diagnostic confirmation within 3 months of age, and 32 (59.26%) by 6 months, as per the national recommendation. In comparison, 4200 newborns were delivered during the post-database integration period, and 4059 (96.64%) received screening before 1 month. A total of 3819 (93.53%) newborns passed the initial screen, whereas 264 (6.47%) were referred. Of those referred, 112 (42.42%) newborns were lost to follow-up and 152 (57.58%) underwent rescreening, leading to 19 (52.78%) newborns completing diagnostic ABR. Among these, 10 (52.63%) newborns were diagnosed by 3 months, meeting the JCIH benchmark, and 16 (84.21%) were diagnosed by 6 months, aligning with the national recommendation. Baseline demographics and clinical risk profiles were similar between cohorts, minimizing the likelihood that population differences contributed to the observed outcomes.

Quantitative comparisons showed significant improvements after database adoption. Screening coverage before 1 month of age increased from 83.47% to 96.64% ($p < 0.001$) (RR 1.16, 95% CI 1.14–1.18), while the referral rate decreased markedly from 18.44% to 6.47% ($p < 0.001$) (RR 0.35, 95% CI 0.31–0.40). Although overall follow-up completion rates did not differ significantly (56.08% vs. 57.58%) ($p = 0.74$) (RR 1.03, 95% CI 0.91–1.16), the proportion of infants completing diagnostic ABR by 3 months increased substantially from 7.41% to 52.63% ($p < 0.001$) (RR 7.11, 95% CI 2.52–20.22). Moreover, the proportion diagnosed by 6 months increased from 59.26% to 84.21% ($p = 0.06$) (RR 1.42, 95% CI 1.06–1.91), meeting the national target and aligning more closely with JCIH benchmarks. These findings demonstrate that database integration enhanced early diagnosis and alignment with JCIH benchmarks, as shown in Figure 2.

Figure 3 shows that a total of 8 children were diagnosed with Sensorineural Hearing Loss (SNHL) in the pre-database integration group compared with 6 children in the post-database group. Unilateral SNHL was observed in 6 cases before integration and 4 cases after, whereas bilateral SNHL remained constant at 2 cases in each group. Hearing aid uptake was limited, with only 1 child in each group receiving amplification, both beyond the recommended 6-month intervention window. The majority of diagnosed children did not receive hearing aids, with 7 cases pre-integration and 5 cases post-integration. These findings indicate that while database integration improved the timeliness of diagnosis, challenges remain in ensuring timely hearing aid fitting and intervention for affected children, as shown in Figure 3.

https://doi.org/10.3390/children13010022

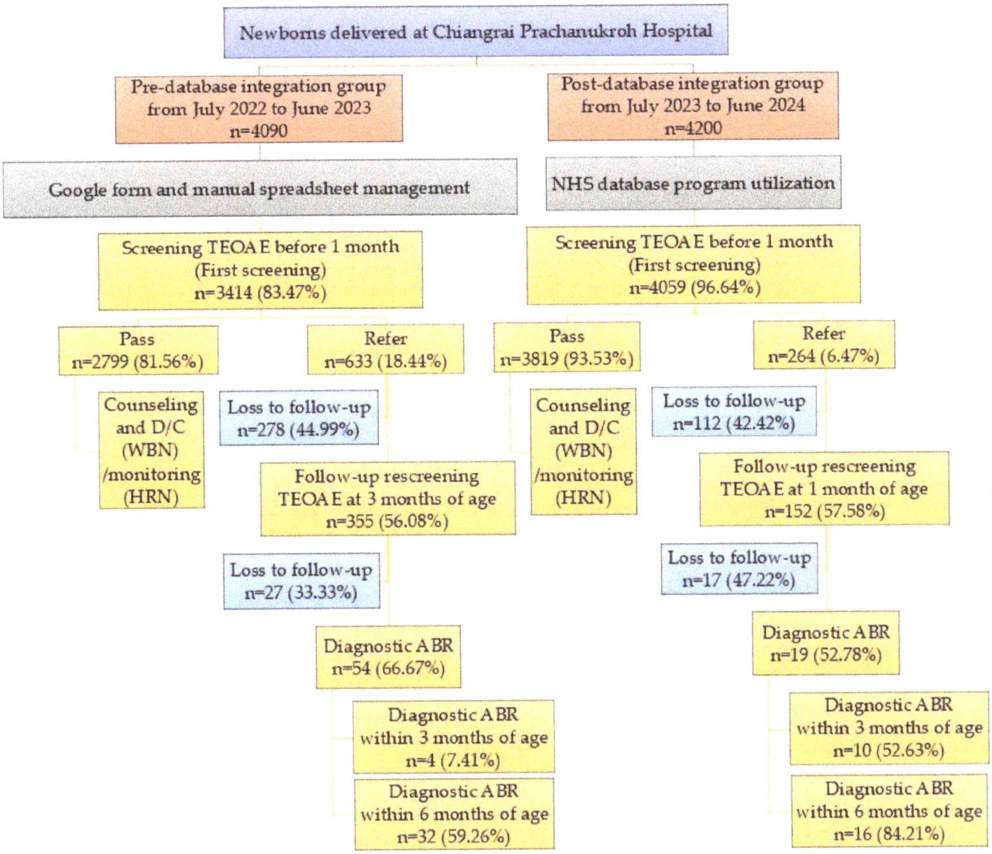

Figure 1. Flow of newborn hearing screening, follow-up, and diagnostic pathways between pre- and post- database integration. Abbreviation: TEOAE, transient evoked otoacoustic emissions; D/C, discharge; WBN, well-baby newborns; HRN, high-risk newborns; ABR, auditory brainstem response. Note: Denominators differ because "screening ≤ 1 month" includes only newborns screened within the first month, whereas pass/referral rates use the total number screened.

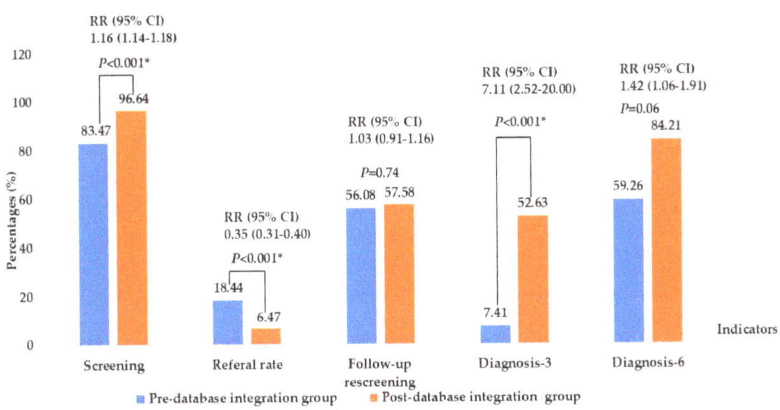

Figure 2. Comparison of key performance indicators of newborn hearing screening between pre- and post- database integration. Note: * Significant at p-value < 0.05; Screening: screening ≤ 1 month of age; Diagnosis-3 and -6: audiological diagnosis ≤ 3 and -6 months of age.

https://doi.org/10.3390/children13010022

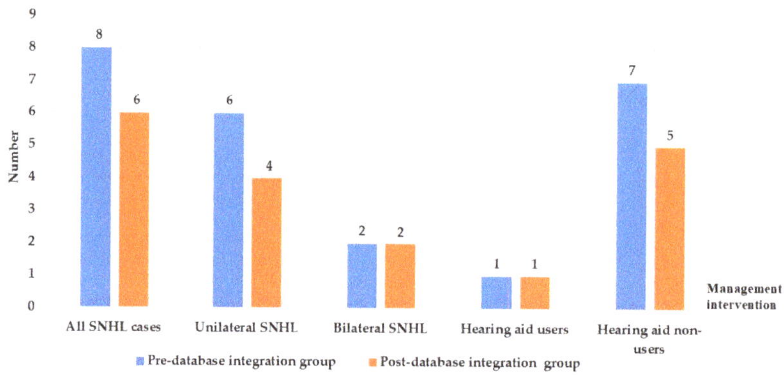

Figure 3. Distribution of SNHL cases and hearing aid management between pre- and post- database integration. Abbreviation: SNHL, sensorineural hearing loss.

4. Discussion

The present study provides one of the first real-world evaluations of hospital-level NHS database integration in a resource-limited setting in Thailand. The findings demonstrate that improvements were observed following database implementation. However, persistent challenges remain in follow-up completion, intervention uptake, and data quality, underscoring the complexity of sustaining EHDI benchmarks in LMICs. Program efficiency and screening outcomes demonstrated measurable improvements following database integration. Integration of the dedicated NHS database yielded clear benefits in workflow management. Screening coverage before one month of age increased statistically significantly from 83.47% to 96.64%, surpassing both national and international benchmarks. This improvement was largely attributable to enhanced workflow coordination and real-time tracking enabled by the NHS database, which reduced missed cases and supported timely screening before discharge [10,11]. However, because this study compared two consecutive 12-month periods without a control group, the observed differences may also reflect temporal changes unrelated to database implementation. Increasing staff experience, periodic refresher training, or concurrent public health activities could have contributed to improved performance across the screening pathway. Interpretation must also consider that Thailand's national NHS algorithm underwent major revisions in July 2023, coinciding with database introduction. The shift from screening within 7 days and rescreening at 3 months to screening within 24–48 h and rescreening at 1 month likely contributed to improvements in first-screen timing. Thus, these outcomes represent the combined effect of national workflow changes and database supported enhancements rather than database impact alone. The referral rate decreased substantially from 18.44% to 6.47% following database implementation. This reduction reflects workflow improvements rather than changes in physiological screening performance, as the database minimized process related errors including incomplete documentation, missed second screenings, and premature refer entries, that previously inflated referral numbers [6,10]. The database did not alter OAE device thresholds or clinical screening protocols but standardized data entry, enabled real-time verification, and ensured that infants requiring repeat screening were correctly identified before being labeled as referrals. These workflow-driven improvements likely reduced false-positive referrals and enhanced accuracy across the screening pathway. Importantly, diagnostic confirmation by three months increased from 7.41% to 52.63%, while confirmation by six months reached 84.21%, approaching the JCIH "1-3-6" target [9,12]. However, interpretation of this improvement must consider concurrent protocol changes. In the post-integration period, the rescreening interval was shortened from approximately

https://doi.org/10.3390/children13010022

three months to one month, which facilitated earlier ABR referral; therefore, the observed gains cannot be attributed solely to database implementation. Interpretation of diagnostic timing also requires caution due to the small and unequal denominators between periods. In the post-database cohort, only 19 infants reached the diagnostic ABR stage, so each case accounted for roughly 5.3% of the overall proportion. As a result, the apparent increase—from four to ten infants diagnosed by three months—produces percentage estimates that are inherently unstable. The reduction in the number of infants requiring ABR (54 to 19) aligns with the markedly lower referral rate (18.44% to 6.47%) and likely reflects improved screening specificity and more efficient rescreening workflows. The analytic approach also imposed limitations. Diagnostic timing was dichotomized ($\leq$3 months vs. >3 months) because assessment dates were recorded categorically rather than as continuous time intervals. Although aligned with JCIH benchmarks, this reduced granularity and may have obscured meaningful variation in diagnostic trajectories. More refined approaches, such as survival analysis or comparisons of median time-to-diagnosis, would yield greater interpretive value if individual-level time data were available. Additionally, multiple screening and diagnostic outcomes were evaluated, increasing the potential for inflated Type I error, although these outcomes represent sequential steps within a single clinical pathway. The NHS database primarily functioned as a workflow-enhancement tool rather than a diagnostic decision system. Its benefits stemmed from structured data entry, improved completeness, automated follow-up list generation, and reduced administrative errors, all of which contributed to more timely screening and diagnostic processes. User feedback indicated that the system was easy to operate after brief training and experienced minimal downtime, supporting feasibility in resource-limited settings. These observations reflect operational characteristics reported during implementation and are therefore presented as interpretative insights rather than quantitative outcomes. Follow-up tracking and diagnostic timeliness showed notable improvements after database integration. Although the overall follow-up completion rate changed only modestly (56.01% vs. 58.46%), the quality and timeliness of follow-up improved, supported by real-time alerts and pre-allocation of ABR diagnostic slots that facilitated earlier evaluation, particularly for high-risk newborns. Prior research at our hospital demonstrated that missed follow-up is largely driven by socioeconomic and geographic barriers, caregiver work demands, long travel distances, forgetting appointments, and low perceived importance of follow-up rather than system limitations [13]. These factors cannot be fully addressed by a database alone, which explains why improved tracking did not produce substantial gains in follow-up completion. Compared with other LMICs reports, in which follow-up loss often exceeds 30–40% [14,15], the relatively stable loss-to-follow-up rate in this study suggests that database integration minimized, but did not eliminate, systemic barriers such as caregiver awareness, transportation, and inter-hospital referral difficulties. International experiences, including the South Korean national database and Dutch regional coordination systems, similarly emphasize that digital integration is necessary but insufficient without concurrent investment in family-centered follow-up and outreach strategies [16,17]. Despite earlier diagnosis, persistent gaps in intervention were evident. Only one child in each cohort received hearing aids, both beyond six months of age, leaving most diagnosed infants untreated. This pattern mirrors other LMICs contexts, where financial constraints, limited device availability, and inadequate rehabilitation pathways delay intervention [18,19]. Review of individual cases showed that delays were primarily caregiver-driven; several families did not return for scheduled fitting appointments despite automated reminders and follow-up calls, resulting in prolonged time to amplification. These findings indicate that improvements in screening workflow alone cannot ensure timely intervention. Structural barriers, including caregiver readiness, financial concerns, logistical constraints, transportation difficulties, low parental

https://doi.org/10.3390/children13010022

awareness, and limited pediatric audiology resources, require targeted strategies beyond database implementation. Several benchmarks traditionally influenced by digital infrastructure, including accuracy of documentation, completeness of rescreening logs, referral tracking, and loss-to-follow-up showed smaller improvements. This pattern suggests that although the database strengthened internal coordination and reduced administrative errors, caregiver-level and socioeconomic factors remain the primary drivers of persistent follow-up challenges. Global EHDI experiences increasingly incorporate tele-audiology and mHealth solutions to address distance and workforce limitations. Tele-diagnostic infant assessments in South Dakota and rural South Africa have demonstrated that remote ABR services are feasible and can expand access for infants who fail initial screening [20]. Recent reviews indicate that remote hearing screening and intervention are non-inferior to traditional pathways and may reduce loss-to-follow-up [21]. mHealth-based hearing-health programs in LMICs further underscore scalable, low-cost approaches for caregiver engagement and follow-up support [22]. Finally, although significant differences were observed between the pre- and post-integration periods, this study was limited to univariate analyses. Incomplete or inconsistently recorded individual-level variables prevented multivariate modeling, limiting our ability to identify independent predictors of outcomes. As a before–after study without a control group, the observed improvements cannot be attributed solely to the database implementation. Changes in screening coverage, referral accuracy, and diagnostic workflow may also reflect temporal trends, increasing staff experience, or other concurrent operational adjustments. Therefore, the findings should be interpreted as correlational rather than causal, as the design does not allow for disentangling database effects from other influencing factors.

The findings highlight how digital transformation in screening workflows can enhance program efficiency, coordination, and diagnostic timeliness while revealing persistent challenges in sustainability and interoperability. The implementation of a dedicated NHS database produced measurable improvements across multiple dimensions of program performance, particularly in workflow efficiency, interdepartmental coordination, and data-driven monitoring. Integration of the NHS database markedly improved workflow efficiency and overall program performance across departments. The centralized data entry system minimized redundant paperwork and manual cross-checking errors, while real-time tracking of screening and follow-up processes allowed healthcare teams to promptly identify missed or delayed cases [23]. Although improvements in workflow efficiency were observed operationally during implementation, workflow efficiency itself was not directly measured as a quantitative outcome. Therefore, these observations should be interpreted as system-level insights rather than data-derived findings. This improvement reflects qualitative observations, as the number of data-entry errors was not quantitatively recorded. Automated scheduling of diagnostic ABR slots and parent reminders enhanced coordination between maternity, pediatric, and audiology units, thereby reducing staff workload and communication gaps. These features collectively facilitated earlier completion of both screening and diagnostic procedures and improved adherence to the JCIH "1-3-6" benchmarks [11]. The database also introduced standardized and structured data fields that strengthened data governance and monitoring capacity. Automatic generation of summary reports and performance dashboards enabled continuous monitoring of screening coverage, referral rates, and diagnostic completion, aligning with both national and international performance indicators. These real-time analytics provided hospital administrators with actionable insights for quality improvement. Similar outcomes have been reported from other digital EHDI platforms in South Korea, Israel, and the Netherlands, where centralized databases were shown to reduce referral rates and accelerate early diagnosis [10,16,17,24]. Unlike systems reported in South Korea or Israel, which primarily serve as centralized reporting tools, the Thai NHS database integrates real-time point-of-care data entry, automated follow-up generation, and diagnostic workflow coordination within a single platform. Its low-cost, intranet-based design and minimal training requirements make it particularly suited to resource-limited provincial hospitals, highlighting the system's unique contribution to LMIC newborn hearing screening models. From a coordination perspective, the integrated referral module allowed seamless communication between primary, secondary, and tertiary hospitals through unified appointment management. Both sending and receiving facilities could track patient status and reschedule appointments instantly, reducing caregiver travel burden and improving follow-up compliance. Given this tiered structure, effective communication and data exchange across hospital levels are essential to support accurate referral pathways, timely rescreening, and completion of diagnostic follow-up for outborn and referred infants. These enhancements were based on qualitative workflow observations, as they were not measured quantitatively. The database supported more equitable access to diagnostic and rehabilitative services across regional networks by standardizing referral workflows and enabling shared, real-time tracking across facilities, thereby reducing geographic disparities and contributing to improved clinical timeliness for high-risk newborns. Furthermore, the system strengthened data governance through multi-level user authorization and encryption protocols that ensured confidentiality and accountability in accordance with Thailand's PDPA. This level of information security represents a critical prerequisite for public trust and large-scale implementation of digital health systems in LMICs.

Despite these improvements, several operational and structural limitations remain. First, data accuracy still relied on staff compliance and manual entry, as automatic validation tools were not embedded in the system. This limitation occasionally resulted in incomplete or inconsistent data fields, reflecting the need for automated verification and standardized operating procedures to enhance data reliability. Second, interoperability with national health information systems and private hospital databases remains limited. The NHS database has not yet been linked to Thailand's HDC, electronic claims system (e-Claim), or other Ministry of Public Health (MOPH) registries. Third, dependence on internet connectivity in rural hospitals posed operational constraints. Network instability delayed real-time data synchronization, particularly in mountainous or remote areas, while smaller hospitals with limited diagnostic resources were unable to fully utilize the system's capabilities. Fourth, persistent loss to follow-up among outborn or high-risk newborns remains a challenge. This limited data exchange hindered long-term tracking of outborn newborns delivered outside the study hospital and referred from external facilities, who often lack unified electronic records and therefore account for a substantial proportion of loss-to-follow-up. Although real-time alerts and tracking improved follow-up for inborn newborns, incomplete inter-hospital data linkage continues to limit continuity of care. This pattern is consistent with global experiences, where even well-designed digital systems cannot fully overcome barriers related to transportation, parental awareness, or socioeconomic constraint [14,15,18,19]. Finally, compliance with PDPA presents ongoing challenges. Although the database incorporates encryption and controlled access, further refinement such as user certification, audit trails, and data anonymization, is needed to ensure full legal compliance and to support national-scale adoption.

For long-term sustainability, the NHS database should evolve toward interoperability with existing MOPH platforms such as the HDC, e-Claim, and other national registries. Seamless integration would enable longitudinal tracking of outborn newborns, reduce data fragmentation, and facilitate continuity of care across provinces. Linking the NHS system with maternal and child health records could also support holistic care pathways that connect hearing screening data with vaccination, growth monitoring, and develop-

https://doi.org/10.3390/children13010022

mental follow-up. Continuous training and technical support are vital to ensure consistent and accurate data entry, particularly in peripheral hospitals where staff turnover is high. Establishing regional "data stewards" or coordinators to oversee data quality and troubleshoot system issues can further strengthen accountability. From a policy perspective, incentive mechanisms such as pay-for-performance (P4P) schemes and recognition-based awards may enhance data accuracy and timeliness, as demonstrated in other digital health programs. Embedding automated error-checking, reminder notifications, and decision-support algorithms could also reduce human error and improve operational efficiency [25]. Integration of tele-audiology such as remote ABR interpretation or virtual counseling would expand access to diagnostic and rehabilitative services in geographically isolated areas [21,25]. Ensuring sustainability requires national-level investment in server maintenance, cybersecurity, and system upgrades. Budget allocation for these components should be incorporated into hospital operational plans and MOPH service frameworks. Collaboration with academic institutions and technology partners can drive continuous innovation while maintaining alignment with national policy priorities. Translating the benefits of database integration into sustainable national outcomes demands a comprehensive policy framework that emphasizes interoperability, human resource development, and continuous quality improvement across all levels of the healthcare system [26]. Ultimately, the NHS database represents a scalable model for digital transformation in early hearing detection and intervention programs in resource-limited settings. Its successful implementation in a provincial hospital demonstrates that structured digital systems can significantly improve screening coverage, diagnostic timeliness, and inter-hospital coordination. However, to achieve national adoption and sustainability, Thailand must strengthen data interoperability, workforce capacity, and system governance. Building on these foundations will ensure that digital innovations translate into measurable, equitable, and enduring improvements in newborn and child health outcomes, in alignment with WHO and JCIH recommendations for universal EHDI [27,28].

This study has several limitations that should be considered when interpreting the findings. First, it was conducted in a single tertiary hospital, which may limit generalizability to other healthcare settings. The retrospective design relied on existing medical records, some of which contained incomplete or inconsistently documented data, particularly during the pre-database period. Although tracking improved for inborn newborns, loss-to-follow-up persisted and was largely driven by caregiver-related barriers such as limited awareness, transportation challenges, and work constraints, factors that the database alone cannot fully address. The post-integration assessment covered only 12 months, which may not adequately reflect long-term system performance or sustainability. Several methodological limitations also warrant attention. Diagnostic timing was dichotomized into ≤3 months versus >3 months due to the absence of uniformly recorded continuous time-to-diagnosis data, resulting in loss of granularity. Multiple comparisons across screening and diagnostic indicators may have increased the potential for Type I error. The absence of a control group restricts causal inference, as improvements may reflect temporal trends, increased staff experience, or concurrent changes in national screening algorithms. Additionally, multivariate analysis could not be performed because individual-level covariates were incomplete or inconsistently recorded; therefore, the results represent unadjusted associations. The database incorporated functions for tracking post-diagnostic intervention; however, timely hearing-aid fitting remained limited by caregiver non-adherence rather than system capacity. Despite automated reminders and follow-up calls, several caregivers did not return for scheduled appointments, resulting in amplification beyond six months in both periods. These observations highlight the need for enhanced family education, counseling, and community outreach to ensure that early detection leads to timely habilitation.

https://doi.org/10.3390/children13010022

Future research should include multicenter studies to evaluate generalizability, longitudinal assessments to examine long-term sustainability, and integration of multivariate or time-series analyses to identify independent predictors of screening and diagnostic outcomes. Evaluating cost-effectiveness, system usability, and interoperability with national health information platforms will also be essential to support large-scale implementation. Strengthening family engagement strategies, exploring mHealth or tele-audiology solutions, and addressing socioeconomic barriers will be critical to translating earlier diagnosis into timely intervention and improved developmental outcomes.

5. Conclusions

The integration of a dedicated NHS database improved screening coverage, referral accuracy, and diagnostic timeliness by strengthening workflow coordination, standardizing data entry, and enabling automated follow-up. However, modest gains in follow-up completion and persistently low hearing-aid uptake indicate that digital workflow enhancements alone cannot overcome caregiver-level socioeconomic barriers or systemic limitations in early intervention services. Because the study used a before–after design without a control group, the observed improvements should be interpreted as associations rather than causal effects. Tele-audiology solutions, including remote ABR interpretation and virtual counseling, offer promising opportunities to expand access in underserved regions and complement database-driven improvements. Sustaining these digital innovations will require national investment in infrastructure, cybersecurity, and interoperability, supported by coordinated planning between hospitals, academic partners, and the Ministry of Public Health. A comprehensive policy framework emphasizing workforce development and continuous quality improvement is essential to translate digital integration into long-term national impact. Future multicenter and longitudinal studies are needed to evaluate generalizability and identify independent predictors of improved outcomes.

Author Contributions: Conceptualization, S.K.I. and K.K.; methodology, K.P., S.K.I., and K.K.; software, K.P. and J.S.; validation, S.K.I. and K.K.; formal analysis, K.P., J.S., and K.K.; investigation, K.P., S.K.I., and K.K.; resources, K.P.; data curation, K.P. and J.S.; writing—original draft preparation, K.P. and K.K.; writing—review and editing, K.P., J.S., S.K.I., and K.K.; visualization, S.K.I. and K.K.; supervision, K.K.; project administration, S.K.I. and K.K.; funding acquisition, K.P. and K.K. All authors have read and agreed to the published version of the manuscript.

Funding: This work was (partially) supported by Research Institute for Health Sciences, Chiang Mai University, grant number 009/2566.

Institutional Review Board Statement: Ethical approval was granted by the Ethical Review Committee for Human Research at Chiangrai Prachanukroh Hospital, under protocol number EC CRH 009/66 In, on 22 June 2023. Participant's consent was waived due to the retrospective study.

Informed Consent Statement: Subject consent was waived due to the retrospective study.

Data Availability Statement: The datasets used and/or analyzed during the current study are available from the corresponding author upon reasonable request.

Acknowledgments: The authors would like to thank staff nurses regarding data collection.

Conflicts of Interest: The authors declare no conflicts of interest in this work.

https://doi.org/10.3390/children13010022

Abbreviations

ABR	Auditory brainstem response
EHDI	Early hearing detection and intervention
LMICs	Low- and middle-income countries
NHS	Newborn hearing screening
TEOAE	Transient evoked otoacoustic emissions
UNHS	Universal newborn hearing screening

References

1. Jariengprasert, C.; Lerdsukprasert, K.; Kasemsuwan, L.; Nannareumitra, P. Universal newborn hearing screening using transient otoacoustic emissions: 1 year prevalence in Ramathibodi hospital. *Thai J. Otolaryngol. Head. Neck Surge* **2003**, *4*, 27–41.
2. Erenberg, A.; Lemons, J.; Sia, C.; Trunkel, D.; Ziring, P. Newborn and infant hearing loss: Detection and intervention.American Academy of Pediatrics. Task Force on Newborn and Infant Hearing, 1998–1999. *Pediatrics* **1999**, *103*, 527–530.
3. Colella-Santos, M.F.; Hein, T.A.; de Souza, G.L.; do Amaral, M.I.; Casali, R.L. Newborn hearing screening and early diagnostic in the NICU. *Biomed. Res. Int.* **2014**, *2014*, 845308. [CrossRef] [PubMed]
4. Reid, A.; Firns, S.; Tao, K.; Maywood, E.; Herbert, H.; Mulders, W.A.M.; Kuthubutheen, J.; Brennan-Jones, C. Early detection of hearing loss for infants in Western Australia: Comparison to international benchmarks. *J. Paediatr. Child. Health* **2022**, *58*, 422–426. [CrossRef] [PubMed]
5. Chouyboonchum, T.; Chamchoi, P.; Chaikhamrongkul, T.; Isarangura, S.; Tiravanitchakul, R. Universal Newborn Hearing Screening and Incidence of Hearing Loss in Ramathibodi Hospital: A 5 Years Experience (2014 to 2018). *RMJ* **2022**, *45*, 25–34.
6. Khaimook, W.; Suwanno, R.; Dindamrongkul, R.; Intusoma, U. An Early Hearing Detection and Intervention Program in Songklanagarind Hospital. *J. Health Sci. Med. Res.* **2022**, *40*, 551–559. [CrossRef]
7. Thongsrinuch, P.; Junthong, S. Prevalence of early hearing detection and intervention newborn in Vajira hospital. *Vajira Med. J.* **2021**, *65*, 39–52.
8. Pitathawatchai, P.; Khaimook, W.; Kirtsreesakul, V. Pilot implementation of newborn hearing screening programme at four hospitals in southern Thailand. *Bull. World Health Organ.* **2019**, *97*, 663–671. [CrossRef]
9. Yimtae, K.; Potaporn, M.; Kaewsiri, S. *The Committee of Newborn Hearing Screening Guidelines of Thailand*, 1st ed.; Off-Set: Bangkok, Thailand, 2019.
10. Chang, J.; Oh, S.H.; Park, S.K. Comparison of newborn hearing screening results between well babies and neonates admitted to the neonatal intensive care unit for more than 5 days: Analysis based on the national database in Korea for 9 years. *PLoS ONE* **2020**, *15*, e0235019. [CrossRef]
11. Mackey, A.R.; Busse, A.M.L.; Del Vecchio, V.; Maki-Torkko, E.; Uhlen, I.M. Protocol and programme factors associated with referral and loss to follow-up from newborn hearing screening: A systematic review. *BMC Pediatr.* **2022**, *22*, 473. [CrossRef]
12. American Academy of Pediatrics, Joint Committee on Infant Hearing. Year 2007 position statement: Principles and guidelines for early hearing detection and intervention programs. *Pediatrics* **2007**, *120*, 898–921. [CrossRef]
13. Parangrit, K. Factors affecting newborn hearing screening follow-up at Otolaryngology Department, Chiangrai Prachanukroh Hospital. *CMJ* **2022**, *14*, 10–17.
14. Bezuidenhout, J.K.; Khoza-Shangase, K.; De Maayer, T.; Strehlau, R. Outcomes of newborn hearing screening at an academic secondary level hospital in Johannesburg, South Africa. *S. Afr. J. Commun. Disord.* **2021**, *68*, e1–e8. [CrossRef] [PubMed]
15. Olusanya, B.O.; Wirz, S.L.; Luxon, L.M. Community-based infant hearing screening for early detection of permanent hearing loss in Lagos, Nigeria: A cross-sectional study. *Bull. World Health Organ.* **2008**, *86*, 956–963. [CrossRef] [PubMed]
16. Park, S.K.; Chang, J.; Im, G.J.; Ahn, J.H.; Lee, J.H.; do Han, K.; Chung, J.W.; Kim, J.S.; Jang, H.; Lee, S.H. Status of early hearing detection and intervention in South Korea: A nationwide population-based study of national infant health checkup. *Sci. Rep.* **2020**, *10*, 16838. [CrossRef]
17. Korver, A.M.; Konings, S.; Dekker, F.W.; Beers, M.; Wever, C.C.; Frijns, J.H.; Oudesluys-Murphy, A.M. Newborn hearing screening vs later hearing screening and developmental outcomes in children with permanent childhood hearing impairment. *JAMA* **2010**, *304*, 1701–1708. [CrossRef]
18. Monica, S.D.; Ramkumar, V.; Krumm, M.; Raman, N.; Nagarajan, R.; Venkatesh, L. School entry level tele-hearing screening in a town in South India—Lessons learnt. *Int. J. Pediatr. Otorhinolaryngol.* **2017**, *92*, 130–135. [CrossRef]
19. Olusanya, B.O.; Newton, V.E. Global burden of childhood hearing impairment and disease control priorities for developing countries. *Lancet* **2007**, *369*, 1314–1317. [CrossRef]
20. Hannah, W.; Riley, E.; Messersmith, J. South Dakota Early Hearing Detection and Intervention Program: Using Teleaudiology to Conduct Infant Diagnostic Assessments. *JEHDI* **2020**, *5*, 47–53.
21. D'Onofrio, K.L.; Zeng, F.G. Tele-Audiology: Current State and Future Directions. *Front. Digit. Health* **2021**, *3*, 788103. [CrossRef]

22. du Plessis, D.; Mahomed-Asmail, F.; le Roux, T.; Graham, M.A.; de Kock, T.; van der Linde, J.; Swanepoel, W. mHealth-Supported Hearing Health Training for Early Childhood Development Practitioners: An Intervention Study. *Int. J. Environ. Res. Public Health* **2022**, *19*, 14228. [PubMed]
23. Parangrit, K.; Sillabutra, J.; Isaradisaikul, S.K.; Kulprachakarn, K. Comparative study of the efficacy between new and routine newborn hearing screening protocols in public hospital, Thailand. *J. Matern. Fetal Neonatal Med.* **2025**, *38*, 2531150. [CrossRef]
24. Wasser, J.; Ari-Even Roth, D.; Herzberg, O.; Lerner-Geva, L.; Rubin, L. Assessing and monitoring the impact of the national newborn hearing screening program in Israel. *Isr. J. Health Policy Res.* **2019**, *8*, 30. [CrossRef]
25. Frosolini, A.; Franz, L.; Caragli, V.; Genovese, E.; de Filippis, C.; Marioni, G. Artificial Intelligence in Audiology: A Scoping Review of Current Applications and Future Directions. *Sensors* **2024**, *24*, 7126. [CrossRef] [PubMed]
26. Lin, M.J.; Chen, C.K. Breaking Sound Barriers: Exploring Tele-Audiology's Impact on Hearing Healthcare. *Diagnostics* **2024**, *14*, 856.
27. WHO. *Hearing Screening Consideration for Implementation*; CC BY-NC-SA 3.0 IGO: Geneva, Switzerland, 2021.
28. American Academy of Pediatrics, Joint Committee on Infant Hearing. Year 2019 position statement: Principles and guidelines for early hearing detection and intervention programs. *Pediatric* **2019**, *4*, 1–44.

https://doi.org/10.3390/children13010022

children

MDPI

Article

Middle Ear Disorders in Children with Down Syndrome: The Detrimental Effect on Speech and Language Development

Ariel Tenenbaum [1,2], Avraham Ben Yaakov [3,†], Yair Peled [1], Malena Cohen-Cymberknoh [1,2], Diana Averbuch [1,2], Ronit Brodie [4] and Menachem Gross [2,3,*,†]

[1] Department of Pediatrics, Hadassah-Hebrew University Medical Center, Jerusalem 91120, Israel; tene@hadassah.org.il (A.T.); yair@peledconsulting.co.il (Y.P.); malena@hadassah.org.il (M.C.-C.); adiana@hadassah.org.il (D.A.)
[2] School of Medicine, Hebrew–University, Jerusalem 91120, Israel
[3] Department of Otolaryngology–Head & Neck Surgery, Hadassah-Hebrew University Medical Center, Jerusalem 91120, Israel; avrahambn@hadassah.org.il
[4] Department of Surgery, Hadassah-Hebrew University Medical Center, Jerusalem 91120, Israel; ronitu@hadassah.org.il
* Correspondence: gross@hadassah.org.il
† These authors contributed equally to this work.

Abstract: Objectives: Our aim was to determine the prevalence of middle ear disorders and associated risk factors that contribute to speech and language developmental delays in children with Down Syndrome. **Methods**: A prospective, cross-sectional study was conducted in 70 children with Down Syndrome between the ages of 1 and 18. Data, including complete physical and otorhinolaryngological examinations, hearing tests, and evaluation of speech and language skills, was compared to a historic typical control group. **Results**: Recurrent otitis media was significantly higher in the study group (56.5%) compared to the control (26%) ($p = 0.05$). The rate of conductive hearing loss was significantly higher in the study group (71.2%) compared to the control (14.9%) ($p = 0.0001$). Conductive hearing loss was statistically associated with delayed speech development ($p = 0.046$). **Conclusions**: Middle ear disorders are common in children with Down Syndrome and are associated with conductive hearing loss and delay of speech and language development. This study emphasizes the importance of routine examination of this population by an Otorhinolaryngologist and speech therapist.

Keywords: down syndrome; otitis media; hearing loss; speech development; middle ear; developmental delay

1. Introduction

Certain otorhinolaryngological (ORL) disorders are known to contribute to cognitive and developmental delay of speech. Among these are hearing impairments, frequently caused by recurrent ear infections or chronic middle ear effusion (CMEE). Children with Down Syndrome (DS) are at increased risk for many ORL illnesses, and as their intellectual capacity is compromised to begin with, the developmental consequences may be particularly grave. Thus, there is great significance for the early identification of ORL disorders in this population.

Children with DS have several predisposing factors that increase the incidence of infections. In addition to an immature immune system, they also have Eustachian tube dysfunction, a contracted nasopharynx, and narrow external auditory canals, conducive to frequent blockage by ear wax [1–3].

Ear infections are not uncommonly accompanied by conductive hearing loss (CHL) [4]. A survey of the frequency of hearing loss in typical children in the United States found it to be relatively high, with 14.9% diagnosed with a hearing impairment, although in most cases, only a minor deficit was detected [5]. In children with DS, the prevalence of hearing loss reaches as high as 38–78% and may be secondary to inadequate treatment of prolonged ear infections [1,6–12]. While hearing loss is a well-known risk factor for speech delay in typical children, the exact effect of hearing impairment on speech development in children with DS is not as clear. This population commonly has a baseline developmental delay, so the contribution of hearing loss is more difficult to determine. In addition to their distinct physical challenges, children with DS struggle with speech and language [13]. These obstacles are typically larger than expected for their degree of intelligence. Difficulties in speech and language have a significant and ultimate negative impact on the communicative skills of subjects with DS [14].

Unlike typical children, CMEE and hearing loss persist as children with DS age; therefore, continued surveillance of otologic and audiological status in these children is recommended. Early hearing loss can delay speech and language milestones in children with DS. Previous research indicates that children with hearing impairments exhibit delays in receptive vocabulary, expressive language, and speech accuracy compared to peers with normal hearing. For instance, children with hearing loss were, on average, seven months delayed in receptive vocabulary and comprehension and 24% less accurate in speech production [15]. Furthermore, a study assessing language outcomes in 41 children with DS found significant differences between those with early hearing loss and those with normal hearing. Children with hearing difficulties scored lower on measures of language expression and comprehension, receptive vocabulary, narrative tasks, and speech accuracy [16].

Assessment of children with DS is often complicated due to the wide spectrum of presenting deficits, making accurate assessment of their communication a difficult task. A balanced assessment consists of a variety of methods, including observations of the child as well as direct interactions in the form of standardized, informal, and dynamic assessments. Depending on the child's age and level of abilities, a variety of assessment measures may be applicable to test DS child in the domains of content (vocabulary), form (grammar/syntax), and use (pragmatic language). For children over 3 years of age whose linguistic abilities are just emerging, a vocabulary inventory was conducted. This allows for comparing children with DS features in their development as compared to typically developing peers. For older, more verbal children who are using words, phrases, and/or sentences to express themselves, adapted standardized measures can be used.

The purpose of this study is to evaluate the prevalence of middle ear disorder in children with DS and to assess its effects on speech development. In addition, this study stresses the importance of ongoing ORL screening in children with DS.

2. Materials and Methods

Participants: Of 100 patients, the data from 70 children with DS who were in the care of the DS Center for Children at a tertiary medical center were retrospectively evaluated for this study over the course of 4 years. Exclusion criteria included patients with incomplete data (missing hearing screening/missing speech evaluations) and patients who withdrew from follow-up at the DS Center. In this multidisciplinary DS care center, children are evaluated by a pediatrician, an ORL specialist, and a speech therapist as part of the general follow-up.

Measures: A complete medical history was recorded for each child, including age, gender, history of gestation and delivery, growth and development, nutrition, and general medical issues. The number of siblings and family history were also recorded. Each child's history of ORL disease was documented, including recurrent otitis media (at least three episodes of acute otitis media (AOM) in a period of 6 months, or four or more episodes in 12 months), CMEE (defined as the presence of middle ear effusion for more than three months' time, occurring at any age on evaluation of the patient), hearing loss, recurrent pharyngotonsillitis, recurrent upper respiratory tract infections, indication for myringotomy or tympanostomy tubes, and any history of hospitalizations or surgeries, particularly adenotonsillectomy.

All children underwent complete physical examination by a pediatrician and an ORL specialist. The assessment was to determine the presence of tympanostomy tubes, signs of inflammation of ear canals and/or pharynx, size of the tongue, enlargement of tonsils, and nasal congestion.

All children were evaluated by two professional, experienced speech clinicians who belong to the DS Center for Children. The speech and language assessment was based on age-appropriate milestones. This evaluation consisted of documentation of specific parameters. History and acquisition of language developmental milestones, which belongs to the language developmental test that evaluates both receptive (understanding) and expressive (speaking) skills, was evaluated by the standardized preschool language scale 5 (PLS-5) (from birth to 7 years). Assessment of speech abilities, particularly the use of complete sentences (expressive language), was also assessed by the PLS-5 test. In addition, expression (expressive language) and comprehension (receptive language) were similarly measured by the PLS-5 test. Furthermore, subjects were evaluated for speech disorders, including stuttering, articulation disturbances, phonemic disorders, and lisps movements. Subjects were evaluated for eating or feeding disorders, including motor examination of the mouth, tongue, teeth, gums, and cheeks. Radiologic evaluation of the swallowing mechanism was completed in cases where necessary. Hearing evaluation included audiometry and tympanometry. For those very young children, hearing was evaluated via behavioral testing and testing via SDT/SRT (speech detection threshold/speech reception threshold) on bone.

2.1. Statistical Analysis

The data were analyzed using descriptive statistical methods. Differences between the study group and historic healthy control groups were analyzed using the χ^2 test for categorical variables [4,5]. The association between categorical variables in the study group was analyzed using the χ^2 test or Fisher's exact test. The association between categorical variables and numeric variables was analyzed using the independent t-test. Statistical significance was accepted at a level of $p \leq 0.05$. Statistical tests were performed using SPSS-25 software.

2.2. Ethical Approval

The study protocol was approved by the Hadassah Medical Center ethics committee (HMO-0507-09 and HMO-0665-17).

3. Results

Demographic characteristics of the study group are presented in Table 1. From an ethnic point of view, the Jewish population was predominant (86%). The mean age of the study group was 6.13 (age range 1–18 years). There were 36 (51.4%) boys and 34 (48.6%) girls. One family failed to cooperate with the interview.

Table 1. Demographic characteristics of the study group.

Parameter		Patients N = 70 (%)
Gender	Male	36 (51.4)
	Female	34 (48.6)
Ethnicity	Jewish	60 (86)
	Arab	10 (14)
Age Group (Yrs)	1–2	17 (24.3)
	3–7	29 (41.4)
	8–18	24 (34.3)
Mean age (Yrs)	6.13	

The prevalence of recurrent otitis media and CHL in the study group as compared to the typical population is shown in Table 2. The rate of recurrent otitis media was significantly higher in the study group (56.5%) compared to typical children in the general population (26%) [4] ($p = 0.05$). The rate of CHL was significantly higher in the study group (71.2%) compared to typical children in the general population (14.9%) [5] ($p = 0.0001$).

Table 2. Prevalence of recurrent otitis media and conductive hearing loss in the study group compared to normal historic healthy control group [4,5].

Child's Condition		Observed Prevalence in Study Group	Expected Prevalence [4,5]	*p* Value
Recurrent otitis media	No	30/69 (43.5%)	74%	$p = 0.05$
	Yes	39/69 (56.5%)	26%	
Conductive hearing loss	No	19/66 (28.8%)	85.1%	$p = 0.0001$
	Yes	47/66 (71.2%)	14.9%	

The association between CHL and recurrent ear infections as well as language development, are demonstrated in Table 3. Recurrent otitis media was statistically associated with CHL ($p = 0.001$). However, no statistically significant association was found between recurrent ear infections and adenoidal enlargement, gender, age group, past hospitalizations, or number of siblings. Speech development was assessed through the use of complete sentences; those who did not speak in complete sentences after three years of age were defined as having a developmental delay. CHL was statistically associated with delayed speech development, as only 38.5% of subjects who had CHL spoke in complete sentences, as compared to 61.5% of subjects with normal hearing ($p = 0.046$).

Table 3. Association between conductive hearing loss and recurrent otitis media and language skills as developmental delay.

	Hearing Loss N (%)		***p* Value**
Recurrent otitis media	No	Yes	
No	14 (73.7%)	13 (27.7%)	$p = 0.001$
Yes	5 (26.3%)	34 (72.3%)	
Language skills	No	Yes	
Syllables to a few words	5 (26.3%)	14 (73.7%)	$p = 0.046$
Complete sentences	8 (61.5%)	5 (38.5%)	

4. Discussion

Children with DS are affected by multiple medical problems, several of which have a negative impact on their cognitive development. The added speech delay resulting from CMEE and CHL raises special concern in light of the pre-existing cognitive challenges inherent to DS.

This study demonstrated a high prevalence of recurrent otitis media in children with DS. It also has shown an increased prevalence of CHL in this population and a significant association with recurrent otitis media and CHL. These findings are all in line with previous studies [1,4]. In our study population, the majority of children with DS and CHL had delayed speech development. With other deficits faced by DS children, it is possible that chronic or recurrent hearing impairment compromises their speech and language learning environment and that a higher degree of hearing loss or prolonged periods of middle ear disorder is associated with poor outcomes on speech and language measures. These findings are consistent with other previous studies, such as those by Roberts et al., who found that language and communication development in children with DS, even with underlying mental delay, can be negatively affected by the presence of CMEE [17]. A retrospective study by Laws and Hall on 41 DS subjects aged 2 to 4 years, investigating the impact of early hearing loss on language outcome, showed significant differences between the group of DS subjects with hearing difficulties and DS subjects with more normal hearing. They concluded that early hearing loss has a significant impact on the speech and language development of children with DS [16]. As such, those authors also concluded that frequent hearing evaluation and screening by speech and language specialist is indeed necessary. Our study results further demonstrate the importance of early evaluation and treatment.

Hearing impairment, specifically conductive hearing loss, is likely to be an additional risk factor for further speech and language delay in DS pediatric subjects. In contrast to typically developing children, children with DS may not have the cognitive capacity to compensate for early hearing loss. Hearing impairment should be considered when managing speech and language deficits in children with DS.

With regard to intervention related to hearing status, the needs are clear: infants and children with DS will benefit from an aggressive treatment for hearing loss associated with middle ear disorder. Balkany, in 1980, identified three goals of such treatment: 1. Normalization of hearing through the insertion of tympanostomy tubes or hearing aids in some cases. 2. Interruption of the cycle of recurrent otitis media with effusion through the use of prophylactic medication. 3. Prevention of chronic ear disease through adequate otologic care [18].

Children with DS have a high prevalence of ORL problems, and when left untreated, these can lead to further morbidity, developmental delay, and impaired quality of life. A concerning trend was noticed in our study population; many of the problems were only first observed when the children arrived at our center—including older children. In our opinion, the various signs of ORL problems may erroneously be perceived by caretakers and under-informed medical professionals as inevitable and untreatable parts of DS when, in fact, ORL problems can be treated effectively.

4.1. Limitations of the Study

The study population consisted of children who were in the care of the Center for Children with DS. These children may not adequately represent the general population of children with DS, as they may come from families with relatively high compliance with medical follow-up and treatment. Alternatively, they may be children whose medical condition is relatively complicated to begin with, in which case they may actually experience more ORL disease than most children with DS. Additionally, the base range of IQ and extent of developmental delays of the children included in the study were not taken into consideration. As such, the significance of the effect of CMEE on such underlying delays was not able to be adequately determined.

4.2. Conclusions

Maintaining a high level of awareness of ORL illnesses in children with DS is imperative. Hearing screening tests should be performed routinely and in accordance with current recommendations [9,10,19]. If the child passes the newborn screening study, rescreen is recommended at 6 months of age for confirmation. In cases of external ear canal stenosis, an interval ear examination by an otolaryngologist every 3 to 6 months is recommended until the tympanic membrane is visualized and tympanometry is applicable. From 1 to 5 years, behavioral audiograms and tympanometry should be performed every 6 months until normal hearing levels are established bilaterally through ear-specific testing (behavioral audiogram or auditory brainstem response (ABR threshold)). External canal and middle ear diseases should be monitored by an otolaryngologist and treated promptly. Conductive hearing loss due to CMEE should treated by ventilation tympanostomy tubes. Conductive hearing loss that cannot treated surgically can be rehabilitated by hearing aids or soft-band with a bone anchoring hearing device (BAHD) until surgical management is suitable. From the age of 5 years, an annual ear-specific audiologic evaluation is recommended.

Effective, timely care for this population can be enhanced by providing follow-up and treatment under one roof by a staff trained to be fully attentive to these unique issues for this patient population. We believe that an extensive evaluation of possible ORL disorders is essential for all children and adults with DS. Furthermore, an experienced and dedicated ORL specialist should be a part of the multidisciplinary medical team that operates a medical center for the DS population. Further prospective studies are required to evaluate the correlation between hearing impairment and speech and language development in DS children.

Author Contributions: Conceptualization: A.T., A.B.Y. and M.G. Methodology: Y.P., A.T., M.G. and M.C.-C. Software: A.B.Y., D.A., R.B., A.T. and Y.P. Formal Analysis: A.T., Y.P., M.G. and M.C.-C. Investigation: Y.P., A.T., D.A. and A.B.Y. Data Curation: Y.P., A.T., D.A., M.C.-C. and A.B.Y. Writing—Original Draft Preparation: A.T., A.B.Y. and M.G. Writing—Review and Editing: R.B., M.G. and A.T. Visualization: R.B., M.G. and A.B.Y. Supervision: A.T. and A.B.Y. Project Administration:

A.T., A.B.Y., M.C.-C., M.G. and R.B. All authors have read and agreed to the published version of the manuscript.

Funding: This research received no external funding.

Institutional Review Board Statement: The study was conducted according to the guidelines of the Declaration of Helsinki and approved by the Institutional Review Board of Hadassah Medical Center, protocol code HMO-0507-09 and HMO-0665-17 on 6 December 2017.

Informed Consent Statement: Because the study is a retrospective study on data from a Down Syndrome multidisciplinary clinic at a tertiary medical center, the IRB approved the study according to the guidelines of the Declaration of Helsinki, with a waiver for informed consent.

Data Availability Statement: The original contributions presented in this study are included in the article. Further inquiries can be directed to the corresponding author.

Conflicts of Interest: The authors declare no conflicts of interest.

References

1. Shott, S.R.; Amin, R.; Chini, B.; Heubi, C.; Hotze, S.; Akers, R. Obstructive sleep apnea: Should all children with Down syndrome be tested? *Arch. Otolaryngol. Head Neck Surg.* **2006**, *132*, 432–435. [CrossRef] [PubMed]
2. Shibahara, Y.; Sando, I. Congenital anomalies of the eustachian tube in Down syndrome. Histopathologic case report. *Ann. Otol. Rhinol. Laryngol.* **1989**, *98 Pt 1*, 543–547. [CrossRef] [PubMed]
3. Keiser, H.; Montague, J.; Wold, D.; Maune, S.; Pattison, D. Hearing loss of Down syndrome adults. *Am. J. Ment. Def.* **1981**, *85*, 467–472.
4. Lanphear, B.P.; Byrd, R.S.; Auinger, P.; Hall, C.B. Increasing prevalence of recurrent otitis media among children in the United States. *Pediatrics* **1997**, *99*, e1. [CrossRef] [PubMed]
5. Niskar, A.S.; Kieszak, S.M.; Holmes, A.; Esteban, E.; Rubin, C.; Brody, D.J. Prevalence of hearing loss among children 6 to 19 years of age: The Third National Health and Nutrition Examination Survey. *JAMA* **1998**, *279*, 1071–1075. [CrossRef] [PubMed]
6. Shott, S.R.; Joseph, A.; Heithaus, D. Hearing loss in children with Down syndrome. *Int. J. Pediatr. Otorhinolaryngol.* **2001**, *61*, 199–205. [CrossRef] [PubMed]
7. Chan, J.; Edman, J.C.; Koltai, P.J. Obstructive sleep apnea in children. *Am. Fam. Physician* **2004**, *69*, 1147–1160. [PubMed]
8. Ng, D.K.; Hui, H.N.; Chan, C.H.; Kwok, K.L.; Chow, P.Y.; Cheung, J.M.; Leung, S.Y. Obstructive sleep apnoea in children with Down syndrome. *Singap. Med. J.* **2006**, *47*, 774–779.
9. AAP issues guidelines on health supervision for children with Down syndrome. *Am. Fam. Physician* **1994**, *50*, 695–697.
10. Davidson, M.A. Primary care for children and adolescents with Down syndrome. *Pediatr. Clin. N. Am.* **2008**, *55*, 1099–1111, xi. [CrossRef] [PubMed]
11. Skotko, B.G.; Macklin, E.A.; Muselli, M.; Voelz, L.; McDonough, M.E.; Davidson, E.; Allareddy, V.; Jayaratne, Y.S.; Bruun, R.; Ching, N.; et al. A predictive model for obstructive sleep apnea and Down syndrome. *Am. J. Med. Genet. A* **2017**, *173*, 889–896. [CrossRef] [PubMed]
12. Manickam, V.; Shott, G.S.; Heithaus, D.; Shott, S.R. Hearing loss in Down Syndrome revisited—15 years later. *Int. J. Pediatr. Otorhinolaryngol.* **2016**, *88*, 203–207. [CrossRef] [PubMed]
13. Næss, K.A.; Lyster, S.A.; Hulme, C.; Melby-Lervåg, M. Language and verbal short-term memory skills in children with Down syndrome: A meta-analytic review. *Res. Dev. Disabil.* **2011**, *32*, 2225–2234. [CrossRef] [PubMed]
14. Meyer, C.; Theodoros, D.; Hickson, L. Management of swallowing and communication difficulties in Down syndrome: A survey of speech-language pathologists. *Int. J. Speech Lang. Pathol.* **2017**, *19*, 87–98. [CrossRef] [PubMed]
15. Hall, A. The impact of hearing loss in children with Down syndrome. *ENT and Audiology News*, 1 May 2015; Volume 24, No. 2.
16. Laws, G.; Hall, A. Early hearing loss and language abilities in children with Down syndrome. *Int. J. Lang. Commun. Disord.* **2014**, *49*, 333–342. [CrossRef] [PubMed]
17. Roberts, J.E.; Price, J.; Malkin, C. Language and communication development in Down syndrome. *Ment. Retard. Dev. Disabil. Res. Rev.* **2007**, *13*, 26–35. [CrossRef] [PubMed]

18. Balkany, T.J. Otologic aspects of Down's syndrome. *Semin. Hear.* **1980**, *1*, 39–47. [CrossRef]
19. Bull, M.J.; Trotter, T.; Santoro, S.L.; Christensen, C.; Grout, R.W.; Council on Genetics; Burke, L.W.; Berry, S.A.; Geleske, T.A.; Holm, I.; et al. Health Supervision for Children and Adolescents with Down Syndrome. *Pediatrics* **2022**, *149*, e2022057010. [CrossRef] [PubMed]

children

MDPI

Review

The Otoacoustic Emissions in the Universal Neonatal Hearing Screening: An Update on Selected Asian States (2005 to 2025)

Stavros Hatzopoulos [1,*], Ludovica Cardinali [2], Piotr Henryk Skarzynski [3,4,5] and Giovanna Zimatore [2,6]

1 Clinic of Audiology & ENT, University of Ferrara, 44122 Ferrara, Italy
2 Department of Life Science, Health, and Health Professions, Link Campus University, 00165 Rome, Italy; l.cardinali@unilink.it (L.C.); giovanna.zimatore@uniecampus.it (G.Z.)
3 Heart Failure and Cardiac Rehabilitation Department, Faculty of Medicine and Dentistry, Medical University of Warsaw, 02-005 Warsaw, Poland; p.skarzynski@inz.waw.pl
4 Institute of Sensory Organs, 05-830 Nadarzyn, Poland
5 World Hearing Center, Department of Teleaudiology and Screening, Institute of Physiology and Pathology of Hearing, 02-042 Warsaw, Poland
6 Department of Theoretical and Applied Sciences Applied Physics, eCampus University, 22060 Novedrate, Italy
* Correspondence: sdh1@unife.it

Abstract

Background: Although significant progress has been made in Neonatal Hearing Screening (NHS) over the past two decades, the available data on Universal Neonatal Hearing Screening (UNHS) practices across Asia remain limited. The aim of this scoping review was therefore twofold: (a) to identify and synthesize the most recent literature (within the past 20 years) concerning NHS/UNHS programs in Asian states, and (b) to summarize evidence on screening procedures, the intervention strategies, and the estimated prevalence of congenital hearing loss (HL), with particular attention to cases of bilateral impairment. **Methods**: In line with previous reports from our group on the screening practices in Europe and in Africa, queries were conducted via the PubMed, Scopus and Google Scholar databases for the time window of 2005–2025. The Mesh terms used were "Otoacoustic Emissions (OAE)", "Universal Neonatal Hearing Screening", "congenital hearing loss", "well babies" and "ASIA", as well as all 50 Asian state names. Only research articles and review papers were considered as good candidates. The standard English language filter was used. **Results**: To maintain homogeneity in terms of state area and population, the studies conducted in China and India were excluded from this report and will be the focus of a dedicated paper. Data from 31 papers were considered, reflecting the neonatal hearing practices of 17 Asian states, of which in 12, UNHS programs are considered mandatory. **Conclusions**: The information on the Asian NHS is limited to a low percentage of Asian states. The available data strongly suggest that audiologists and other hearing professionals, involved in regional or national screening initiatives, should collect systematically and disseminate the screening information through peer-reviewed scientific publications. The latter will contribute to a broader understanding of program effectiveness and will facilitate international benchmarking.

Keywords: Asia; congenital hearing loss; newborn hearing screening; otoacoustic emissions; well babies; NICU; bilateral hearing loss

1. Introduction

The goal of any Neonatal Hearing Screening (NHS), or of an Early Hearing Detection and Intervention (EHDI) protocol, is to identify infants who may present sensorineural and conductive hearing impairments. Data from the literature clearly suggest that language development and the relative development of social and cognitive abilities depend on the early identification and rehabilitation of hearing impairments [1,2]. Universal NHS (UNHS) can now be performed using two assessment protocols, based on Otoacoustic Emissions (OAEs) and the Automated Auditory Brainstem Responses (AABRs) [3,4]. Previously reported data in the literature provide the essential information regarding the effects of hearing screening on language development and the inner workings of the now-established clinical screening techniques [5].

OAEs are a rapid, non-invasive, and economical method. Certain brief stimuli (such as clicks, chirps, and tone bursts) are produced by microphones in a tiny probe, which is placed into the newborn's ear canal, and they evoked responses from the cochlea, recorded by the same microphones. Applications for this type of technology are numerous, and they extend as well into the adult population, including the detection of noise-induced hearing loss (HL) or age-related hearing impairment [6]. Most importantly, the data in the literature suggest that OAE hearing screening protocols can detect hearing impairment significantly earlier than the traditional pure tone audiometry assessment [7].

As we have previously reported in the analysis of the NHS European [8] and African data [9,10], NHS programs appear to encounter numerous implementation challenges, even though hearing screening is regarded as a necessary clinical practice.

This scoping review focuses on the NHS practices of a number of Asian countries and follows the guidelines we have established in the previous publications. The present work addresses five key questions: (i) Which states have implemented UNHS programs? (ii) What proportion of newborns are screened? (iii) What is the prevalence of congenital, particularly the bilateral, hearing loss (HL)? (iv) If reported, what are the follow-up rates? and (v) Which screening protocols and OAE technologies are most commonly employed?

2. Materials and Methods

We sourced scientific articles using the PubMed, Scopus, and Google Scholar search engines. As in the previous reviews, we have selected a 20-year time window (2005–2025) to address existing informational gaps. Baseline data were derived from the comprehensive, survey-based study by Neumann [11] in 2020, which analyzed healthcare systems across 196 states worldwide.

Asia accounted for approximately 4.8 billion inhabitants in 2024 [12], encompassing countries with markedly diverse demographic, healthcare, and regulatory characteristics. For methodological reasons, studies conducted in China and India were excluded from the present review. These two countries represent exceptional cases within the Asian region, owing to their extremely large populations, highly heterogeneous healthcare infrastructures, and the long-standing implementation of independently developed newborn hearing screening programs. Inclusion of China and India would have disproportionately influenced the synthesis and limited the comparability of findings across countries with smaller populations and more homogeneous regulatory frameworks. The present review, therefore, focuses on Asian countries with broadly comparable programmatic and contextual characteristics, while evidence from China and India will be addressed in a separate forthcoming manuscript. The assessed Asian states (in bold) as shown in Table A1 in Appendix A.

The search of the literature was carried out in September 2025 in accordance with the PRISMA 2020 framework (website accessed 4 July 2025, the check list is reported in Supplementary Materials). Three primary MeSH terms guided the selection process:

https://doi.org/10.3390/children13010060

"OAE," "Neonatal Hearing Screening," "congenital hearing loss," and "Asia" or the name of each Asian state. Only English-language research articles were included (reviews and single or sporadic case reports were not considered), while studies dealing with NHS outside Asia were excluded.

Selection quality was ensured by prioritizing publications in peer-reviewed journals. Preference was also given to studies presenting transparent methodologies and a consistent application of established screening protocols.

The inclusion criteria for the review were established as follows: (i) the geographical affiliation of the study (Asian origin versus other regions); (ii) the size of the screened population, with preference given to larger cohorts; and (iii) the recency of data, selecting the most up-to-date study or studies available for each country.

References were drawn from PubMed, Scopus, and Google Scholar. Two independent reviewers assessed the retrieved material, resulting in a final selection of 48 eligible papers. A second screening excluded 17 papers for geographic origin in China and India. The PRISMA flow diagram is presented in Figure 1, while the studies included in the review are summarized in Table 1.

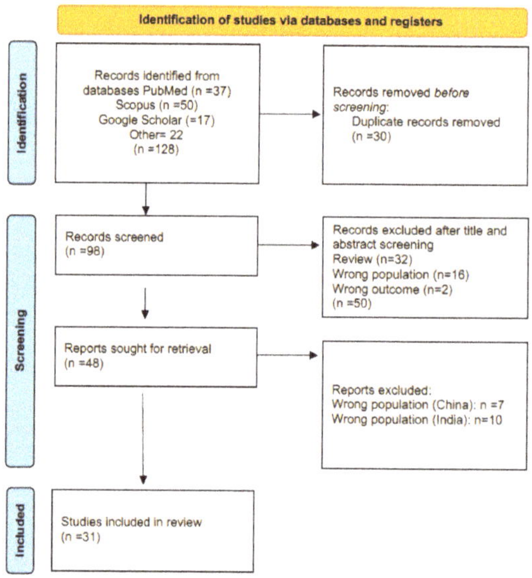

Figure 1. Flow diagram of literature search, according to PRISMA criteria (https://www.prisma-statement.org/prisma-2020, accessed 4 July 2025), with the steps followed in the manuscript selection procedure. After the application of the selection criteria, the initial 128 manuscripts were reduced to 31.

Table 1. The 31 eligible papers after the filtering process are as follows. The data are presented in alphabetical order for each state; NA = Not Available Information; NICU, Neonatal Intensive Care Unit; NHS, Neonatal Hearing Screening).

n	State	Region/City or Town	Sample Size (n)	Study Period	Authors (First Name)	Publication Year
1	Indonesia	Surabaya	60	2023	Falerina [13]	2023
2	Iran	Southwestern	92,521	March 2013–April 2016	Saki [14]	2017
3	Israel	Ziv Medical Center	5496 (5212)	Mar 2010–Dec 2011	Gilbey [15]	2013
4		Beer-Sheva	238	2024	Ziv [16]	2024
5		NA	5621	2014–2023	Farladansky-Gershnabel [17]	2025
6	Japan	Okayama	47,346	2001–2005	Fukushima [18]	2008

https://doi.org/10.3390/children13010060

Table 1. *Cont.*

n	State	Region/City or Town	Sample Size (n)	Study Period	Authors (First Name)	Publication Year
7		Akita	35,461	2012–2016	Sato [19]	2020
8	Jordan	Amman	416	2024	Qanawati [20]	2024
9	Malaysia	Kuala	2713 (NICU)	2014–2016	Abdullah [21]	2020
10		Kuala, Sarawak, Kedah, Perak	58,862 (28,432 + 30,340)	2015–2016	Wong [22]	2021
11	Nepal	Kathmandu	5517	2015–2016	Shrestha [23]	2017
12	Oman	Al-Seeb	12,743	2016–2018	Kolethekkat [24]	2020
13	Pakistan	Karachi	267	2020–2021	Pyarali [25]	2023
14	Philippines	Manila	NA	2009 -	Labra [26]	2023
15	Saudi Arabia	Jeddah	11,986	1996–2004	Habib [27]	2005
16		Riyadh	20,171	2016	Alanazi [28]	2020
17		Riyadh	130 (children)	2025	Elbeltagy [29]	2025
18	Singapore	Singapore	100,225	2002–2009	Jayagobi [30]	2019
19		Singapore	29,972	2004–2014	Tang [31]	2022
20	South Korea	Seoul	43	NA	Kim [32]	2013
21		Seoul	185 children (109 NHS data)	2008–2017	Lee [33]	2019
22	Syria	Refugees in Turkey	6034	2018	Kaplama [34]	2020
23	Taiwan	Taiwan	1017	2011	Wu [35]	2011
24	Thailand	Bangkok	507 high-risk infants	2005 (18-month study)	Srisuparp [36]	2005
25		Northern	3120 (infants at 3 months)	Nov 2010–May 2012	Poonual [37]	2015
26		Northern	3120 (development evaluation from 6 to 18 months)	Nov 2010–May 2012	Poonual [38]	2017a
27		Northern	3120	Nov 2010–May 2012	Poonual [39]	2017b
28		Southern	6140	January–July 2017	Pitathawatchai [40]	2019
29	Turkey	Izmir	711	2007	Tatli [41]	2007
30		Ankara	16,975	Jan 2007–Feb 2008	Tasci [42]	2010
31		Istanbul	4111 healthy; 1874 high-risk	2016	Yılmazer [43]	2016
32		Sanliurfa	37,219	01–12/2018	Kaplama [34]	2020

3. Results

The data extracted from the 31 selected studies were classified alphabetically according to the state of origin, and the information obtained is summarized in Table 2.

Table 2. Data presenting the various Asian NHS national activities. The national data are presented in alphabetical order. The second column presents the NHS protocols used. The third column reports the overall HL prevalence, or the bilateral and unilateral HL estimates, when calculated or reported. The fourth column reports the major causes of HL as reported by the corresponding publication. The last two columns refer to the first author and the year of the relevant publication. Abbreviations: OAEs: Otoacoustic Emissions; TEOAE: Transient-Evoked OAE; DPOAE: Distortion Product OAE; AABR: Automated Auditory Brainstem Response; ABR: Auditory Brainstem Response; ASSR: Auditory Steady State Response; SNHL: Sensorineural Hearing Loss; CHL: Conductive Hearing Loss; MHL: Mixed Hearing Loss; CI: Cochlear Implant; HL: Hearing Loss; LBW: Low Birth Weight; UNHS: Universal Newborn Hearing Screening; PTA: Pure Tone Average; bil. HL: Bilateral HL; uni. HL: Unilateral HL. #: sample is too small to generalize; NA = Not Available Information.

State	Screening Protocol (OAE/ABR)	Hearing Loss Prevalence	Causes/Risk Factors	Author (First)	Year
Indonesia	DPOAE at >24 h, 1 and 2 months; ABR for persistent REFER cases	2/60 #	Prematurity, LBW, low Apgar; most improved after serial testing	Falerina [13]	2023

https://doi.org/10.3390/children13010060

Table 2. *Cont.*

State	Screening Protocol (OAE/ABR)	Hearing Loss Prevalence	Causes/Risk Factors	Author (First)	Year
Iran	Two-stage TEOAE + AABR; diagnostic ABR/OAE at ≤3 mo	bil. HL (1.52/1000) uni. HL (0.89/1000)	87% sensorineural, 12.5% auditory neuropathy; higher rural referral	Saki [14]	2017
Israel	TEOAE + AABR; high-risk infants	7/5212 1.3/1000 Estimate is optimistic since, for significant number of REFERs, testing was not possible	NA	Gilbey [15]	2013
	OAE + ABR (UNHS); post-UNHS cohort analysis	238 children with confirmed HL Initial sample size is NOT reported	Consanguinity is associated with higher bilateral HL and delayed/poor CI compliance	Ziv [16]	2024
	TEOAE within 48–72 h after birth	NA	Cesarean section and vacuum-assisted deliveries increased false-positive risk (OR 7–15×)	Farladansky-Gershnabel [17]	2025
Japan	Two-stage AABR + clinical ABR follow-up for 24 months	bil. HL (108/47,346) uni. HL (140/47,346) 5.2/1000	NA	Fukushima [18]	2008
	Two-stage AABR + clinical ABR or ASSR	bil. HL (47/33,547) uni. HL (97/33,547) 4.3/1000	For 1 bil. HL cases, mutation of Gap-junction beta-2 protein was found	Sato [19]	2020
Jordan	DPOAE + ABR	77.9% with HL (65% SNHL; 33% CHL; 1% MHL) #	Strong association with consanguineous marriage (38.46%) and family history	Qanawati [20]	2024
Malaysia	OAE (not specified) + AABR + clinical ABR	15.36/1000	Craniofacial anomalies were the factor most related to HL; Infants with 3 or more risk factors presented 100% HL	Abdullah [21]	2020
	DPOAE+ AABR	3.15/1000	NA	Wong [22]	2021
Nepal	Two-stage ABR (birth + 6 weeks); diagnostic ABR for persistent REFER	Apparent 6.7% (374/5517 referred); higher among NICU infants (9%) #	Risk factors: LBW, prematurity, ototoxic drugs, hyperbilirubinemia, mechanical ventilation	Shrestha [23]	2017
Oman	Two-stage TEOEA + Clinical ABR	3.37/1000	Craniofacial complications and syndromic HL	Kolethekkat [24]	2020
Pakistan	Two-OAE stages (protocol not specified) + clinical ABR.	18/267 HL #	Gestational age, craniofacial abnormalities	Pyarali [25]	2023
Philippines	Two-stage testing + Clinical ABR/ASSR	NA	NA	Labra [26]	2016
Saudi Arabia	Two-stage TEOAE (<48 h + day 5) + diagnostic ABR	0.18% HL; 0.17% bil. SNHL	Congenital bil. SNHL dominant (20/22)	Habib [27]	2005
	PTA + TEOAE + Tympanometry (school-age follow-up)	0.17–0.18% congenital bil. HL; 5.4% prevalence of delayed onset	Consanguinity increases risk of late SNHL	Alanazi [28]	2025
	Two-stage TEOAE (<48 h, <2 weeks)	referral rate: 1.33%	NA	Elbeltagy [29]	2020
Singapore	Two-stage AABR	35/1000 overall 19.9/1000 permanent HL	Craniofacial anomalies, mechanical ventilation > 5 days auditory neuropathy incidence 1.1/1000	Jayagobi [30]	2020
	Two-stage TEOAE+ AABR	117/29,671 or 3.9/1000	NA	Tang [31]	2023
South Korea	ABR (majority), TEOAE (minority); confirmatory ABR/ASSR	NA	Biallelic SLC26A4 (PDS) mutations; late diagnosis	Kim [32]	2013
	TEOAE + ABR; In case of REFER confirmation by ABR + ASSR	NA	SLC26A4 (PDS) mutations (41% in NHS-pass group); later diagnosis in NHS-referred group	Lee [33]	2009

https://doi.org/10.3390/children13010060

Table 2. *Cont.*

State	Screening Protocol (OAE/ABR)	Hearing Loss Prevalence	Causes/Risk Factors	Author (First)	Year
Syria	Two-stage TEOAE + AABR	26/6034 or 4.3/1000.	17 (65.4%) presented risk factors as n days NICU stay, hyperbilirubinemia, consanguineous marriage, and family history of HL.	Kaplama [34]	2020
Taiwan	Two-stage DPOAE + genetic screening (GJB2, SLC26A4, m.1555A > G) + ABR	Hearing screening referral rate: 3.7%	Genetic causes could not be identified by UNHL	Wu [35]	2011
Thailand	Automated OAE/ABR (AccuScreen) in high-risk infants	Bil. HL 4.1% uni. HL 2.6% 6.7/1000	Risk factors: craniofacial anomalies, mechanical ventilation > 5 days	Srisuparp [36]	2005
	Two-stage TEOAE + ABR (prospective cohort study, infant at 3 months)	135/3120 or 43/1000 (very high value)	Risk factors independently associated with bilateral HL (birth weight, craniofacial anomalies, sepsis and ototoxic exposure)	Poonual [37]	2015
	Evaluation following the Two-stage TEOAE + ABR from 6 to 18 months (analytic prospective study)	14/3120 or 4.48/1000	Risk factors: ototoxic exposure, low APGAR, craniofacial anomalies (see details in Table 5 of [38])	Poonual [38]	2017a
	Two-stage TEOAE + ABR; risk prediction via COBRA score	43/1000	Risk factors COBRA score: (craniofacial anomaly, ototoxicity, birth weight, relative history, Apgar); 80% of existing HR was detected	Poonual [39]	2017b
	OAE (TEOAE) two-stage + ABR; confirmation speech development at 12 months	12/5859 or 2.04/1000	Assisted ventilation, ototoxic drugs, duration in NICU, syndromic HL	Pitathawatchai [40]	2019
Turkey	Two-stage TEOAE + ABR (diagnostic)	1.21/1000	SNHL predominant	Tatli [41]	2007
	Two-stage TEOAE + ABR (diagnostic)	bil. HL (28/16,975), uni. HL (10/16,975) 2.2/1000	Ototoxic drugs (39.5%), NICU stay > 7 days, prematurity (39.5%)	Tasci [42]	2010
	Two-stage TEOAE + ABR (diagnostic)	bil. HL (8/5985) uni. HL (3/5985) 1.8/1000	(60%) prolonged mechanical ventilation or neonatal intensive care, (50%) consanguineous marriage, (10%) LBW, (10%) family history of HI and (10%) hyperbilirubinemia.	Yılmazer [43]	2016
	Two-stage TEOAE + AABR	84/37,219 or 2.26/1000.	35 (65.4%) risk factors such as n days NICU stay, hyperbilirubinemia, consanguineous marriage, family history of HL	Kaplama [34]	2020

3.1. Indonesia

Zislavsky et al. [44] coordinated a multicenter study in Indonesia on the factors associated with the time of diagnosis and habilitation of congenital HL. They reported in 2023 that the estimated prevalence of congenital HL in Indonesia was a high value of approximately 110/1000, showing an increasing pattern from the reported value of 80/1000 in 2013.

In terms of NHS, a prospective study conducted by Falerina et al. [13] at Dr. Soetomo General Academic Hospital in Surabaya evaluated the feasibility and outcomes of newborn hearing screening using Distortion Product OAEs (DPOAEs). Although no national UNHS policy was in place (in the year 2023), this investigation represents one of the few structured implementations of serial hearing screening in the country, with the downside of a rather small sample size. A total of 60 neonates were enrolled, equally divided between those with (n = 30) and without (n = 30) risk factors for HL. Screening was conducted universally within the hospital setting, using DPOAEs at three time points: >24 h after birth, 1 month, and 2 months of age. Infants who continued to yield REFER results after the third session were referred for Auditory Brainstem Response (ABR) testing. Across

https://doi.org/10.3390/children13010060

the three sequential screenings, the proportion of infants screened reached 100% of those born in the study hospital. The pass rate improved markedly from 18% at >24 h, to 36% at 1 month, and 96% at 2 months, demonstrating the effectiveness of serial screening in reducing false positives. Only two infants (3.3%), one with prematurity and one with low birth weight (LBW), retained REFER outcomes after the final screening and were referred for confirmatory ABR evaluation. This represents an apparent prevalence of suspected congenital HL of approximately 3% (a rather high estimate), although no confirmed ABR results were reported.

Follow-up adherence across the three test sessions was excellent, with all 60 newborns completing the screening sequence. The study highlights that DPOAE technology is feasible, cost-effective, and adaptable to resource-limited Indonesian hospital settings. The authors recommend serial universal screening at birth, 1 month, and 2 months to reduce unnecessary referrals and ensure early detection before 6 months of age.

3.2. Iran

Saki et al. [14] evaluated 92,521 newborns (46,147 boys and 46,374 girls) between March 2013 and April 2016, from the Khuzestan Province (southwestern Iran) as part of a national UNHS initiative, covering virtually 100% of eligible live births in the region (67,780 urban; 24,741 rural). A two-stage protocol combining Transient-Evoked OAEs (TEOAEs) and Automated ABR was used: first within 48 h after birth, repeated at ≤1 month, and with full diagnostic ABR/OAE evaluation by ≤3 months for persistent REFER cases. The coverage rate approached 100%, with a 4.2% loss to follow-up (LTF).

Confirmed HL was diagnosed in 223 infants, corresponding to a prevalence of 2.41 per 1000 live births. Of these, 141 infants (1.52 per 1000) presented bilateral HL and 82 infants (0.89 per 1000) unilateral impairment. Most cases (87%) were sensorineural, 12.5% were auditory neuropathy, and a small minority were conductive losses (5%). Severe-to-profound degrees of loss predominated, with no significant sex difference ($p = 0.29$). Of the 10,804 neonates who required rescreening, 4.23% (457 infants) were lost to follow-up. Among those who completed the second stage, 98.75% of all screened newborns ultimately passed, leaving 1.25% (1161) referred for full diagnostic evaluation. Follow-up compliance was generally high, though slightly lower in rural settings due to limited audiological resources and travel barriers. The combined TEOAE + AABR strategy effectively minimized false positives and captured auditory neuropathy cases, providing outcomes comparable to high-income states.

3.3. Israel

Israel has fully implemented a UNHS program, mandated by the Ministry of Health since January 2010. The program requires that all newborns be screened before hospital discharge, reflecting one of the most comprehensive and well-organized early hearing detection systems in the Middle East. The program combines OAE testing and ABR to ensure early detection of congenital and neural hearing disorders, including auditory neuropathy. Three complementary studies described the national screening outcomes in Israel.

Gilbey et al. [15] analyzed 5496 live births at Ziv Medical Center (Zefat). A two-stage TEOAE + AABR protocol achieved 94.8% coverage, 5.2% referral, and 70–81% diagnostic follow-up by the age of three months. In total, 34 infants were diagnosed with hearing impairment (27 conductive, 7 mild–moderate sensorineural).

Ziv et al. [16] examined 238 children diagnosed with hearing impairment post-UNHS. Among those born from consanguineous unions, bilateral HL and delayed or incomplete compliance with cochlear implantation were significantly more frequent. The authors of the paper comment that Israeli UNHS programs reach a >95% national coverage by applying

https://doi.org/10.3390/children13010060

TEOAE + AABR protocols, though sociocultural factors such as consanguinity still affect long-term outcomes and follow-up compliance.

In 2025, Farladansky-Gershnabel et al. [17] reported data from 5621 infants with normal hearing, identifying 6.5% false-positive OAE results. Cesarean section and vacuum-assisted deliveries were significant predictors of false-positive outcomes (OR ≈ 7–15 vs. vaginal delivery), underscoring the influence of perinatal factors on screening accuracy.

3.4. Japan

The first pilot NHS study was conducted in the Okayama prefecture from 2001 to 2005, and Fukushima et al. [18] reported the data in 2008. According to the authors, 47,346 infants (corresponding to a coverage of 95%) were screened with AABR and followed for 24 months. From this sample, 248 neonates presented a hearing impairment (108 bilateral HL and 140 unilateral HL). Three cases who initially passed the AABR test were later (the time is not specified) diagnosed with a late-onset HL. The authors also comment that the screening protocol of the pilot study was carefully designed to work with the Japanese societal trends (not specified), suggesting that societal factors are equally important in NHS strategies to the actual screening protocols selected.

In 2020, Sato et al. [19] published data from the Akita region, using a time frame of 5 years and achieving the second largest assessed NHS sample in Japan. From 2012 to 2016, 35,461 infants were screened via a two-stage AABR, resulting in a coverage rate of 94,7%. The AABR protocol was the same as in the Fukushima et al. study, where a two-stage AABR was used to identify HL. REFER cases from the first AABR were retested one day before discharge. The REFER cases from the second stage were diagnosed with a clinical ABR within a timeframe of 3 months. The authors reported that 179 infants were identified with a probable HL and were sent to the otorhinolaryngology department of the collaborating hospitals for a final diagnosis. Of those, 36 were not included in the assessment. The identified HL cases included 47 with bilateral deficits, 55 with a right-ear and 42 with a left-ear HL. The overall incidence of HL reported was 144/33,545 = 4.3/1000. Genetic testing was also conducted on the bilateral HL cases to identify the possible causes of the congenital HL. Only one infant was identified with a mutation of the Cap-junction beta-2 protein.

3.5. Jordan

Recent studies in Jordan have focused not only on screening implementation but also on identifying key genetic and demographic determinants of congenital and early childhood HL.

The most recent and comprehensive data come from Qanawati et al. [20], who investigated the relationship between consanguineous marriage and HL in Jordanian children. The authors conducted a retrospective analysis between 2020 and 2023 of 416 pediatric patients (<18 years) at the Al-Ahliyya Amman University Hearing and Speech Center. Screening and diagnostic methods included DPOAEs, ABR, and pure-tone audiometry, indicating adherence to established early detection protocols. In the analyzed cohort, 77.9% (n = 324) of children were diagnosed with HL, with a predominance of sensorineural HL (SNHL; 65%), followed by conductive (33%) and mixed (1%) types. The mean age of onset was 5 months, reflecting early detection consistent with neonatal or infantile origin. While the study did not explicitly differentiate between congenital and acquired etiologies, the findings underscore a high burden of early-onset and likely genetic HL within the Jordanian pediatric population. Logistic regression revealed that children from consanguineous marriages had significantly higher odds of HL (log odds = 0.895; $p = 0.029$), particularly

https://doi.org/10.3390/children13010060

for sensorineural and mixed types, and that family history acted as a compounding factor (interaction term $p = 0.007$).

3.6. Malaysia

Abdullah et al. [21] reported HL data from neonatal residents of the Intensive Care Unit (NICU) in a Kuala-Lampur tertiary hospital. The authors assessed data from 2713 infants from January 2014 to December 2016. The tested protocol consisted of OAEs and AABR (the type of OAEs was not specified). 214 Infants who resulted as REFER by both screening procedures were tested by a clinical ABR within a time frame of 30–90 days. From those, the final assessment was possible only for 105, and in this group, 40 neonates were diagnosed with a HL. In total, 32 presented a bilateral HL, 7 presented a right-ear unilateral HL and 1 presented a left-ear unilateral HL. The estimated incidence of HL was 40/(2713-109 who did not complete the final ABR) = 15.36/1000, a rather high value. From the considered risk factors only, craniofacial anomalies were found to be significantly related to HL. For infants presenting three or more risk factors, the probability of having a hearing impairment was 100%.

Wong et al. [22] reported the results of a retrospective analysis on UNHS data from four public Malaysian hospitals in the time frame of 2015 and 2016. The authors have presented their data in terms of each year to show the progress achieved from one year to another. In this review, the data have been pooled together. A total of 58,862 infants were assessed with a mean regional coverage of 81.2%. The screening protocol consisted of a first stage conducted with DPOAEs and the second with AABR. According to the authors, "Depending on hospital resources, automated AABR and DPOAE were used, either alone or combined, as the hearing screening tool". The total number of infants diagnosed with a hearing impairment was 186, suggesting an HL incidence of 3.15/1000. In terms of quality measures, the study data showed that " The return for follow-up rates for each participating hospital was generally below the recommended benchmark of 95%" [45]. The mean age at screening was 3.9 days and 3.3 days, respectively, for the years 2015 and 2016, showing an improvement in the age of identification. From the 186 infants who presented HL, the mean age for the 70 infants diagnosed with a permanent HL was 4.7 ± 0.7 months in 2015 and 3.6 ± 0.9 months in 2016, both below the expected 6-month intervention limit.

3.7. Nepal

The study by Shrestha et al. [23] at Dhulikhel Hospital, Kathmandu University Hospital, represents the first large-scale prospective implementation of UNHS in Nepal.

The Dhulikhel Hospital program began in February 2017 as a structured pilot of universal screening for all inborn infants and those admitted to the Neonatal Intensive Care Unit (NICU). The study demonstrated that a two-stage Automated ABR protocol can be successfully implemented. During the study period (February 2017–October 2019), 5517 of 5956 live births (92.6%) were screened. Of these, 422 (7.7%) were NICU infants and 5095 (92.3%) were well babies. In the first-stage screening, 30% of well babies and 35% of NICU babies were referred ("REFER"). In the second-stage rescreening (after 6 weeks), referral rates dropped to 6.6% among well babies and 9.0% among NICU babies. The overall referral rate after the second screening was 6.7% (374/5517), demonstrating the value of a two-step process in reducing false-positive results. The prevalence of confirmed congenital HL was not directly reported, as diagnostic follow-up ABR outcomes were beyond the study's scope. However, using referral as a proxy indicator, the apparent prevalence of suspected congenital HL was approximately 6.7% overall and higher in NICU infants (9%) compared to well babies (6.6%). Among the risk factors analyzed, LBW and prematurity were the most frequent, followed by ototoxic drug exposure, hyperbilirubinemia, and mechanical ventilation. Follow-up compliance was high: all infants who failed the first screening

https://doi.org/10.3390/children13010060

were scheduled for rescreening at 6 weeks, coinciding with immunization visits. The integration with vaccination schedules minimized attrition, resulting in nearly complete follow-up across both well and sick newborns. The authors emphasized that this combined health-service approach is feasible and sustainable for national scale-up.

3.8. Oman

Abdullah et al. [24] reported data from a retrospective review conducted from January 2016 to December 2018 in a tertiary hospital in Oman. A sample of 12,743 infants was assessed, and the reported regional coverage was 90%, dropping to 88.4% for the second screening stage. The testing protocol consisted of a two-stage TEOAEs followed by a clinical ABR for the resulting REFER cases. In total, 43 infants were diagnosed with HL, 29 presented a bilateral HL and 11 presented with unilateral losses. The estimated HL incidence for this sample was 43/12,743 = 3.37/1000. In terms of risk factors, significant relationships with HL were found for craniofacial anomalies and syndromic illness. The authors reported relatively long times for the final HL confirmation for the two TEOAE stages as 7.98 and 17.3 weeks, respectively.

For 13 infants of the 43 identified with HL, some sort of early intervention strategy was applied (the authors mention amplification, probably intending the use of hearing aids). The paper also examined the factors which have caused a low return rate, and they commented, "More than 60% of the participants felt that the long waiting period and/or delay in obtaining appointments were the key reasons for the delay in receiving early intervention, and a significant number of them missed appointments as they were not reminded on time". The latter clearly suggests that emerging UNHS programs need a very systematic patient administration, especially after the initial HL identification (intervention phase)

3.9. Pakistan

Pyarali et al. [25] conducted a small prospective cross-sectional study in a Karachi hospital, from November 2020 to April 2021, assessing all born infants in that timeframe. 267 infants were tested with a double-stage OAE protocol (not specified by the authors). In total, 18 infants resulted in REFER and were evaluated by a clinical ABR. Of those, 10 were found with a bilateral HL and 8 with a unilateral HL. For the 42 NICU residents, the following risk factors were identified as important contributors to the observed HL: ototoxic medications (by the mother), radiation exposure (of the mother), permanence in the NICU (days), gestational age and low APGAR score.

The authors make a series of interesting comments regarding the crucial elements of UNHS: (i) they describe their poor experience with LTF (Loss to Follow) for 10 infants, who were identified with a bilateral HL, where only 3 returned for the additional medical checking. Additionally, they discuss some other important factors related to LTF (who were also encountered in a number of African states [9]) in the following: "It is important to discuss with the parents, their failure to understand the importance of screening as well as the early intervention and the need for collaboration between parents and service providers. Other reasons included the lack of transport as they were living in small villages and cities, lack of interest as the family was not prepared for further testing because of financial issues, lack of awareness about early HL identification, social and cultural stigma related to deafness, and negative parental attitude towards hearing screening protocol".

3.10. Philippines

In 2016, Labra et al. [26] conducted a survey on the implementation of UNHS in the Philippines, across 51 newborn hearing screening centers in 12 regions, to assess their compliance with screening protocols, staffing, IT capabilities, and access to specialists. Unfortunately, the paper does not provide any "raw numbers" in terms of the actual

https://doi.org/10.3390/children13010060

infants screened and who and how many have received a hearing intervention. Although important data is missing, the paper provides useful peripheral information on the UNHS practices in the Philippines. The data reported can be grouped into the following:

- From the available centers, 96.1% had certified personnel.
- Only 41.67% of surveyed regions had centers offering confirmatory testing and early intervention services.
- Access to specialists was limited, with only 39.2% of centers having clinical audiologists and 23.5% having speech-language pathologists.
- Assessment was performed initially via a two-stage OAE protocol and then by a clinical ABR/ASSR to verify infants with a suspected hearing deficit.
- Data management was a major issue, with only 3.9% of centers using the online registry and 5.9% using registry cards.
- Internet access was available in 58.8% of centers, but data submission methods were largely non-compliant.
- Patient follow-up systems were inadequate, with only 27.5% of centers tracking newborns referred for confirmatory testing.

The study highlights deficiencies in confirmatory testing, early intervention services, and data management, emphasizing the need for regional centers, improved IT systems, and better resource allocation. Recommendations include decentralizing program management, streamlining registry card procurement, enhancing training and certification processes, and involving pediatricians and community health workers in the program.

3.11. Saudi Arabian Emirates

Three studies published between 2005 and 2025 describe the gradual development and refinement of the UNHS programs in Saudi Arabia and demonstrate the country's transition from early hospital-based initiatives to a near-comprehensive national screening system.

Habib & Abdelgaffar [27] conducted one of the earliest prospective NHS studies at King Fahd Hospital, Jeddah. A total of 11,986 newborns were screened using a two-stage TEOAE protocol performed within 48 h of birth and repeated at 5 days of life for initial REFER cases. At the first screening, 91.3% of newborns passed bilaterally, while 8.7% (n = 1042) were referred for repeat testing. After the second-stage OAE, 0.62% (n = 74) remained REFER. Diagnostic ABR testing at 5 months confirmed 22 cases of SNHL (0.18%), of which 20 were bilateral (0.17%) and 2 unilateral (0.02%). The false-positive rate was reduced from 8.7% to 0.62% after the two-stage design. Parental compliance with follow-up reached 95%, reflecting high acceptance of screening. The authors concluded that the TEOAE-based two-stage program was feasible, accurate, and cost-effective, suitable for integration into public health hospitals nationwide.

Alanazi et al. [28] reported a retrospective cross-sectional descriptive study of national UNHS program data collected from multiple hospitals across Saudi Arabia between 2016 and 2019. Their study described the outcomes of an expanded national-level implementation that utilized automated OAE and AABR technologies in parallel, depending on institutional availability. Across all regions, screening coverage exceeded 90% of live births, with an overall referral rate of 2.8% after the first test and 1.1% after rescreening. The prevalence of confirmed congenital HL was approximately 1.8 per 1000 live births, comparable to global averages. The authors reported persistent challenges related to loss to follow-up cases, averaging 10–12% nationally and recommended the digital centralization of screening data and mandatory follow-up pathways to improve coverage consistency across regions. The findings confirmed that Saudi Arabia's national screening outcomes parallel the data from European and North American programs [8,11,24], reflecting substantial progress in the NHS infrastructure and early diagnosis.

https://doi.org/10.3390/children13010060

Elbeltagy et al. [29] performed a cross-sectional follow-up study assessing 130 children aged 6–7 years who had previously passed newborn hearing screening. Using pure-tone audiometry (PTA), tympanometry, and TEOAEs, the authors identified seven children (5.4%) with delayed-onset bilateral SNHL. Parental consanguinity was present in 71% of the affected group versus 34% in the control group, representing a statistically significant association ($p = 0.026$, OR = 2.6). None of the affected children had previously experienced otitis media or ototoxic exposure, suggesting a predominantly genetic etiology. The study highlights the importance of post-UNHS surveillance for delayed onset and progressive forms of HL, particularly in populations with high consanguinity rates. The authors recommend periodic audiological screening during early school years to capture late-onset SNHL cases that escape neonatal detection.

The combined information from these studies suggests that Saudi Arabia has developed one of the most comprehensive UNHS infrastructures in the Middle East. The two-stage TEOAE protocol remains the foundational approach, now complemented by AABR confirmation and digital reporting. The prevalence of congenital bilateral HL has stabilized around 0.17–0.18%, while delayed-onset HL affects an additional 5% of school-aged children. The primary etiological factor remains genetic consanguinity, highlighting the need for continued family counseling, long-term follow-up, and the inclusion of molecular genetic testing in national EHDI protocols.

3.12. Singapore

Jayagobi et al. [30] reported data on the screening of NICU residents in a tertiary care center, from April 2002 to December 2009. 2906 NICU infants were assessed with an OAE-ABR protocol, and the data were registered within the HITRACK management system. The average age of diagnosis was reported as 4.5 months. Of the 92 infants presenting with HL, 89 had multiple risk factors. The overall incidence of HL for any type and severity was found to be 35/1000, and the rate of congenital permanent HL was 15.4/1000. During additional tests on the infants who passed the first screening after 3–6 months, 12 infants were identified with a permanent late-onset HL, modifying the HL incidence to 19.9/1000. The auditory neuropathy incidence was estimated as 1.1/1000.

Tang et al. [31] presented data from a UNHS program within a time frame of 10 years. A sample of 29,972 infants was assessed with TEOAEs and AABR; 301 infants were found to be non-eligible (deceased or transferred to another hospital). NICU residents were tested with both protocols. A total of 157 infants were referred to a clinical ABR evaluation, but due to incomplete data, only 147 REFER cases were included in the study. Of those, 117 were found with HL. The estimated incidence of HL was reported as 117/29,671 = 3.94/1000. In terms of intervention policies, only 74 infants received assistance, raising, unfortunately, the loss to follow-up value to 35% (41/117). For two cases, the families refused any post-screening intervention.

3.13. South Korea

Two key studies conducted in South Korea have critically examined the performance and limitations of UNHS, particularly in detecting delayed-onset or genetically mediated forms of HL. Both investigations highlighted that conventional screening methods, based on OAEs and AABR, may fail to identify a subset of infants who develop significant hearing impairment later in childhood.

Kim et al. [32] evaluated 43 patients with sensorineural HL carrying biallelic SLC26A4 mutations, a genetic defect associated with Pendred syndrome and enlarged vestibular aqueduct (EVA). In total, 14 of these children had undergone newborn hearing screening. Among them, four infants (28.6%) passed the screening bilaterally, while six (42.9%) passed

https://doi.org/10.3390/children13010060

in one ear and failed in the other. Only four were correctly identified as REFER in both ears. For comparison, among 15 children without SLC26A4 mutations, only 2 (13.3%) passed the screening bilaterally. The average age at which bilateral HL was confirmed in the PASS group was approximately 31.5 months, compared with only 1.7 months in those who had been identified as REFER at birth. This significant diagnostic delay underscored the limitation of the OAE- and the AABR-based screening in detecting infants predisposed to progressive or late-onset HL due to genetic causes. The authors concluded that universal newborn hearing screening alone is insufficient in such cases and recommended the addition of molecular genetic testing, particularly for SLC26A4, to improve early identification of at-risk infants.

Lee et al. [33] further examined the clinical implications of these findings by analyzing a cohort of children who had undergone cochlear implantation after initially passing newborn screening. Among 109 children with available NHS data, approximately 22% had passed the screening at birth but subsequently developed profound bilateral HL necessitating cochlear implantation. In these children, the mean age at diagnosis of HL was 28 months, significantly later than the average of three months in those who had failed the neonatal screen. The study confirmed that progressive or late-onset HL is not uncommon among children who initially PASS NHS, especially those with genetic etiologies such as SLC26A4 or GJB2 mutations. The authors emphasized that current screening protocols cannot detect these cases and advocated for post-neonatal audiological surveillance to ensure early diagnosis and intervention.

The combination of the data derived from these two studies demonstrates that while the national UNHS system successfully identifies most congenital and bilateral cases, it fails to detect a proportion of infants with genetically determined, progressive forms of HL. The evidence suggests that integrating genetic testing with newborn screening and establishing longitudinal audiological monitoring could markedly enhance early detection and improve long-term auditory and language outcomes in this population.

3.14. Syria

There are no reported studies in the literature on any NHS program in Syria, but a Turkish study by Kaplama et al. [34] in the city of Sanliurfa (close to the Syrian border) reports data on a comparison between Syrian (refugees) and Turkish newborns. Considering the absence of other relevant information on the Syrian NHS, it was decided to include this paper in order to present the NHS characteristics of the neonatal Syrian population (born in Turkey).

From January 2018 to December 2018, 6034 Syrian infants were assessed with a two-stage TEOAE protocol followed, if necessary, by an AABR and, in case of another REFER, by a clinical ABR. 34 infants were admitted to a clinical ABR assessment, and 26 were found with a hearing impairment, resulting in an incidence of HL 26/6034 = 4.3/1000. There were no risk factors in 9 (34.6%) of the Syrian newborns with HL, while 17 (65.4%) presented risk factors such as the number of days in the NICU, consanguineous marriage, hyperbilirubinemia and family history of HL.

3.15. Taiwan

Wu et al. [35] implemented a combined DPOAE + newborn genetic screening (NGS) program in 1017 infants at National Taiwan University Hospital. DPOAE was performed at 48 h and repeated before discharge, while blood samples were screened for GJB2, SLC26A4, and m.1555AG mutations. Infants with REFER OAE results or pathogenic genotypes underwent confirmatory ABR by three months. This dual-screening model successfully identified infants with subclinical or at-risk genetic variants, suggesting that integrating NGS with UNHS enhances the detection of progressive or late-onset HL.

https://doi.org/10.3390/children13010060

3.16. Thailand

Five studies conducted in Thailand between 2005 and 2019 tested universal and targeted NHS programs, representing both tertiary and primary care settings.

Srisuparp et al. [36] evaluated a high-risk neonatal screening program at Siriraj Hospital in Bangkok, using an automated combined OAE/ABR device (AccuScreen) operated by trained nurses. Among 507 high-risk neonates, 6.7% (n = 34) had abnormal screening results, including 4.1% bilateral and 2.6% unilateral failures. Univariate analysis using a Chi-square test and multiple logistic regression analysis were used for identification of significant risk factors: independent risk factors for abnormal screening outcomes included craniofacial anomalies (≈42-fold) and mechanical ventilation > 5 days (≈4-fold). The median screening age was 19 days, and nearly all infants (97.3%) were screened before 3 months of age, confirming the feasibility of such a nurse-led program in resource-limited contexts.

Poonual et al. [37] implemented a three-step universal screening protocol at three tertiary hospitals in Northern Thailand using automated OAEs, conventional OAEs, and ABR. Among 3120 infants aged 3 months, 4.3% failed the OAE screening, and 5 (0.16%) were confirmed by ABR with a bilateral SNHL. Major risk factors for HL included LBW, low Apgar score, craniofacial anomalies, sepsis, and ototoxic drug exposure.

Poonual et al. [38] evaluated the outcomes of early identification and development of speech and auditory skills in the same cohort as in [37]. Of 3120 newborns screened by two-stage TEOAE + AABR, 7.5% failed the TEOAE and 4.3% failed the AABR test. At 6 months, 3.3% were diagnosed with congenital HL, though only 0.4% had permanent HL at 18 months. Early intervention before 6 months improved auditory and speech outcomes in all cases, though language development remained delayed in the majority. Major associated risk factors were craniofacial anomalies, ototoxic exposure, hyperbilirubinemia, low Apgar score, and sepsis.

On the same 3120 newborns of the two previous papers [37,38], Poonual et al. [39] proposed the COBRA score (by considering 5 risk factors: Craniofacial anomaly, ototoxicity, birth weight, relative history, Apgar score) as a simple clinical tool for predicting HL risk in primary care. Applied to the same Northern Thai cohort (n = 3120), the COBRA score, derived from multivariable Poisson risk regression, achieved an Area under ROC of 0.95, comparable to the JCIH risk criteria, and correctly identified all infants with confirmed HL (4.3% at 3 months by ABR). This approach was considered suitable for low-resource or primary care environments.

Pitathawatchai et al. [40] conducted a hospital-based program consisting of two stages of OAEs and one stage of ABR on a total of 6140 eligible newborns. Reported bilateral HL prevalence ranged between 0.2 and 0.3% (≈2–3 per 1000 births) with >80–90% follow-up completion, demonstrating high feasibility and national scalability. In total, 12 cases resulted in HL and were enrolled in an early intervention program. Nine of those infants presented normal speech development at 12 months. Data on the total costs of an UNHS program were also reported, with a total expenditure of 8944 USD for every infant diagnosed with sensorineural HL.

In summary, these five studies indicate that Thailand has successfully implemented multi-stage OAE/ABR-based NHS local programs since the early 2000s, achieving high coverage, early diagnosis, and improved outcomes with low false-positive rates. Integration of risk-based scoring systems such as COBRA could further enhance screening in peripheral health settings.

https://doi.org/10.3390/children13010060

3.17. Turkey

Four studies conducted between 2007 and 2020 evaluated the implementation and performance of UNHS programs in Turkey, documenting a steady improvement in screening coverage, diagnostic accuracy, and follow-up adherence over time.

Tatli et al. [41] investigated the feasibility of NHS at a tertiary-level hospital in İzmir. The program used a two-stage protocol consisting of TEOAEs at 48 h postnatal age, followed by diagnostic ABR testing for infants who failed the initial screen. Out of 711 screened newborns, 1.2% (n = 9) were referred for diagnostic assessment, and 0.14% (1/711) were confirmed to have bilateral SNHL. The refer rate after the first TEOAE test was 3.7%, dropping to 1.2% after rescreening. The study demonstrated a 100% parental compliance for follow-up and concluded that NHS is feasible, rapid, and cost-effective even in non-university public hospitals. The authors emphasized that integration into routine postnatal care is key for national expansion.

Tasci et al. [42] conducted a large-scale prospective study in Ankara to evaluate the effectiveness of a two-stage OAE + ABR screening protocol across multiple hospitals. A total of 16,975 neonates were screened between January 2007 and February 2008.

The first-stage OAE REFER rate was 4.9%, reduced to 1.8% after repeat testing. Diagnostic ABR confirmed permanent congenital HL in 31 infants (0.18%), of which 22 (0.13%) were bilateral. The study identified LBW, NICU admission, and family history of HL as significant predictors of permanent HL. The authors concluded that a two-step OAE protocol followed by diagnostic ABR is an efficient, high-yield strategy for national implementation and recommended the creation of regional data registries to monitor screening performance.

Yılmazer et al. [43] analyzed 5985 newborns from two large hospitals in Istanbul (4111 healthy and 1874 high-risk infants) to assess follow-up outcomes and risk factors after newborn hearing screening. The program followed a two-phase model: all well babies (WB) were tested by TEOAEs, while ABR was used for the NICU residents or the WB REFER cases. The initial REFER rate was 4.2% among WB and 10.3% in the high-risk group. The overall hearing-loss prevalence was 1.8 per 1000 live births (11 infants total), of which 8 were bilateral. Parental compliance with diagnostic ABR follow-up was 87%. Among risk factors, prolonged NICU stay, hyperbilirubinemia, and ototoxic medication exposure were the strongest predictors of abnormal OAE results. The authors reported that integrating ABR into the second stage significantly reduced false-positive rates and increased the detection of auditory neuropathy cases. The study concluded that the Turkish national UNHS program had reached levels of quality comparable to those in European states, emphasizing the importance of standardized data recording and ongoing monitoring.

Kaplama et al. [34] in the previously mentioned paper on the Syrian infants, assessed data from 37,219 Turkish neonates with a two-stage TEOAE protocol followed, if necessary, by an AABR and in case of another REFER by a clinical ABR. In total, 132 infants were admitted to a clinical ABR assessment, and 84 were found with a hearing impairment, resulting in an incidence of HL 84/37,219 = 2.26/1000. There were no risk factors in 49 of the newborns with HL, while 35 (65.4%) presented risk factors such as the number of days in the NICU, hyperbilirubinemia, consanguineous marriage, and family history of HL.

Overall, these four Turkish studies highlight the progressive success of Turkey's nationwide UNHS rollout, achieving screening coverage > 90%, follow-up rates > 85%, and a confirmed bilateral HL prevalence between 0.13% and 0.22%. The TEOAE + ABR two-stage protocol remains the national standard, demonstrating high diagnostic reliability, cost-effectiveness, and strong public compliance.

https://doi.org/10.3390/children13010060

4. Discussion

The serious implications of a delayed detection of hearing impairment in the language development of the infant population have been presented and discussed in our previous reviews on NHS practices in Europe [8] and in Africa [9,10]. The objectives of this scoping review were the evaluation of the available NHS data in the Asian states and of any possible updates since the last reported estimates in 2020 by Neumann et al. [9]. In terms of updates, 15 out of the 31 papers used in this review were published from 2020 onwards. In Sections 4.1–4.5 will be reported data aggregated in five key areas targeting the five questions presented in the Introduction Section.

4.1. States Implementing NHS-UNHS Programs

Based on the reviewed evidence, UNHS programs have been implemented either nationally or regionally in multiple Asian and Middle Eastern states, including Indonesia, Iran, Israel, Jordan, Japan, Nepal, Philippines, Singapore, South Korea, Saudi Arabia, Taiwan, Thailand, and Turkey. The level of implementation varies widely: while states such as Israel, South Korea, Thailand, and Turkey have achieved a near-universal national coverage, others, including Indonesia, Jordan, and Nepal, are still developing regional or more often hospital-based screening initiatives. The latter was found to be the established starting-point for any NHS experience, as also observed in numerous African states [9,10].

4.2. Proportion of Newborns Screened

The reported NHS coverage ranged from 60 to 95%, with several national programs reporting near-complete participation. Iran and Israel achieved coverage above 94%, while Saudi Arabia, Thailand, and Turkey reported rates exceeding 90% of live births. In contrast, Indonesia and Nepal presented lower coverage levels, primarily due to resource limitations and decentralized health systems. Importantly, even in states with high coverage, disparities persist between urban and rural or low-resource areas, suggesting that infrastructure and workforce training remain essential to ensure equitable access. Several studies have reported screening on older infants aged 3 months [37] or even children [29].

The data on the follow-up rates (after the initial NHS start-up) varied considerably among the Asian states. Programs with centralized data systems and parental counselling, such as those in Iran, Israel, Saudi Arabia, and Turkey, achieved 85–95% follow-up compliance, comparable to European high-income states [6]. Conversely, LTF numbers remained a major challenge in the low-resource settings like Indonesia and Nepal, where LTF rates exceeded 10–15% in some reports. Consistent parental education, integration of screening data into national registries, and mandatory follow-up pathways were repeatedly identified as critical components for improving post-screening adherence.

4.3. Prevalence of Congenital and Bilateral HL

When reported, the prevalence of congenital HL ranged between 0.1% and 0.4% (1–4 per 1000 live births), values which align with the global NHS standards. Bilateral SNHL was consistently the predominant form, typically accounting for 70–90% of confirmed cases. High reported HL prevalences were seen in the datasets from Malaysia (15.3/1000), Singapore (15/1000) and Thailand (43/1000), but in order to achieve more objective estimates, much larger samples of neonates must be assessed. Notably, states with high rates of consanguineous marriages (Jordan, Saudi Arabia, and parts of Israel) exhibited increased prevalence and delayed-onset cases, underscoring the genetic contribution to pediatric HL in these populations.

https://doi.org/10.3390/children13010060

4.4. Causes Leading to HL and Intervention Strategies

Very few studies have reported the probable causes of HL, including the standard risk factors (days in the NICU, ototoxic drugs, Low birth weight, family history, etc.) and the issue of consanguinity (which was also a significant factor in the reported African HL data).

A total of 3 studies (2 from North Korea and 1 from Taiwan) from the pool of 31 manuscripts provided information on Neonatal Genetic Screening, especially about mutations of the GJB2 and SLC26A4 genes. The reported findings are alarming since they show that infants passing the OAE + AABR tests can be positive for GJB2 or SLC26A4 mutations. These data confirm similar findings from Russia reported in a previous scoping review on the European data [6]. In this context, NHS protocols should be accompanied by an NGS to detect cases probably prone to progressive or late-onset HL.

4.5. Screening Protocols and OAE Technologies

Most states adopted the standard two- or three-stage screening models, by using in the first one- or two-stages the OAEs, followed by a clinical ABR for the OAE REFER cases or the assessment of NICU infants (in UNHS programs). This OAE-ABR combination minimized false-positive results and allowed detection of auditory neuropathy spectrum disorders.

Indonesia demonstrated that serial OAE testing at three time-points, at birth, at 1 month, and at 2 months, can effectively reduce the false referrals in resource-limited settings. Thailand and Turkey have standardized the use of a TEOAE + ABR protocol, while Japan and Taiwan additionally integrate genetic testing (e.g., GJB2, SLC26A4) to identify infants at risk for progressive or late-onset HL.

Emerging strategies, such as the COBRA risk score developed in Thailand, offer practical screening tools for primary care environments with limited technology and based on risk factors independently associated with HL.

4.6. Possible Limitations of the Study

We have identified three areas where the information from the current manuscript might be incomplete:

(i) As in our previous scoping reviews, some limitations might arise from the fact that available and probably significant screening data (for any state in question) are not reported in established impact factor sources and therefore cannot be utilized.
(ii) The pool of papers in this scoping review does not present sufficient information about the intervention strategies applied; once an HL case has been identified, therefore, it was not possible to report in depth any intervention activities. This aspect is quite common in the majority of programs and has also been noted in European and African NHS publications.
(iii) China and India were not included in the review because across these huge states, the sociopolitical gradient and the relative health policies change significantly. Our initial hypothesis was that these data could bias he overall Asian NHS report. A future manuscript will examine the NHS status of these two states.

4.7. Future Directions

From 2005 to 2025, OAEs have remained a cornerstone of UNHS across Asia. Programs that pair OAEs with rescreening, clear diagnostic referral pathways (AABR/ABR), and robust follow-up systems show better program performance [35]. Key priorities for the next decade are reducing the loss to follow-up index with digital registries, validating low-cost portable OAE devices, and producing multi-site comparative evidence to guide regionally appropriate protocols and policy.

5. Conclusions

The data from the literature indicate that many Asian middle-income states have successfully transitioned from pilot hospital-based projects to sustainable UNHS programs, achieving international standards. The overall evidence supports the feasibility and cost-effectiveness of UNHS programs across diverse socioeconomic contexts, provided that screening is accompanied by consistent follow-up, parent engagement, and appropriate referral systems. Fragmented database systems (primarily from local NHS experiences) seem to delay a more nationwide NHS organization.

Supplementary Materials: The following supporting information can be downloaded at: https://www.mdpi.com/article/10.3390/children13010060/s1, Table S1: PRISMA 2020 Checklist [46].

Author Contributions: Bibliographic search, S.H., G.Z. and L.C.; investigation, data curation: S.H., G.Z. and L.C.; writing—original draft preparation, S.H. and G.Z.; writing—review and editing, S.H., G.Z. and P.H.S. All authors have read and agreed to the published version of the manuscript.

Funding: This research received no external funding.

Institutional Review Board Statement: Not applicable.

Informed Consent Statement: Not applicable.

Data Availability Statement: The original contributions presented in this study are included in the article. Further inquiries can be directed to the corresponding author.

Conflicts of Interest: The authors declare no conflicts of interest.

Abbreviations

AABR	Automated Auditory Brainstem Response
ABR	Auditory Brainstem Response
ASSR	Auditory Steady State Response
BD	Bilateral Deafness
CHL	Conductive Hearing Loss
CI	Cochlear Implant
DPOAE	Distortion Product OAE
EDHI	Early Hearing Detection and Intervention
ENT	Ear, Nose, and Throat
HL	Hearing Loss
LBW	Low Birth Weight
LTF	Loss to Follow-Up
MHL	Mixed Hearing Loss
NHS	Neonatal Hearing Screening
NICU	Neonatal Intensive Care Unit
OAEs	Otoacoustic Emissions
PTA	Pure Tone Average
SNHL	Sensorineural Hearing Loss
TEOAE	Transient-Evoked OAE
UNHS	Universal Neonatal Hearing Screening

Appendix A

The Asian continent is composed of 50 states. In various contexts, Asia is divided into five subregions (Central, Eastern, Southern, Southeastern, and Western Asia) [12]. In this review, we have considered the whole continent without any specific geographical divisions. Asia accounts for approximately 59–60% of the world's population and about 30% of the Earth's total land area.

https://doi.org/10.3390/children13010060

Table A1. Assessed states (in bold) for the presence of NHS activities. Data from China and India (in shaded cells) were not considered in the review.

ID	Country	Population	Studies Selected	Region
1	Afghanistan	43,844,111	-	South Asia
2	Armenia	2,952,365	-	Western Asia
3	Azerbaijan	10,397,713	-	Western Asia
4	Bahrain	1,643,332	-	Western Asia
5	Bangladesh	175,686,899	-	South Asia
6	Bhutan	796,682	-	South Asia
7	Brunei	466,330	-	Southeast Asia
8	Cambodia	17,847,982	-	Southeast Asia
9	**China**	**1,416,096,094**	-	**East Asia**
10	China Hong Kong		-	East Asia
11	China Macao			East Asia
12	Cyprus	1,370,754	-	Western Asia
13	Georgia	3,806,671	-	Western Asia
14	**India**	**1,463,865,525**	-	**South Asia**
15	**Indonesia**	**285,721,236**	1	**Southeast Asia**
16	**Iran**	**92,417,681**	1	**South Asia**
17	Iraq	47,020,774	-	Western Asia
18	**Israel**	**9,517,181**	3	**Western Asia**
19	**Japan**	**123,103,479**	2	**East Asia**
20	**Jordan**	**11,520,684**	1	**Western Asia**
21	Kazakhstan	20,843,754	-	Central Asia
22	Kuwait	5,026,078	-	Western Asia
23	Kyrgyzstan	7,295,034	-	Central Asia
24	Laos	7,873,046	-	Southeast Asia
25	Lebanon	5,849,421	-	Western Asia
26	**Malaysia**	**35,977,838**	2	**Southeast Asia**
27	Maldives	529,676	-	South Asia
28	Mongolia	3,517,100	-	East Asia
29	Myanmar	54,850,648	-	Southeast Asia
30	**Nepal**	**29,618,118**	1	**South Asia**
31	North Korea	26,571,036	-	East Asia
32	**Oman**	**5,494,691**	1	**Western Asia**
33	**Pakistan**	**255,219,554**	1	**South Asia**
34	Palestine	5,589,623	-	Western Asia
35	**Philippines**	**116,786,962**	1	**Southeast Asia**
36	Qatar	3,115,889	-	Western Asia
37	**Saudi Arabia**	**34,566,328**	3	**Western Asia**
38	**Singapore**	**5,870,750**	2	**Southeast Asia**
39	**South Korea**	**51,667,029**	2	**East Asia**
40	Sri Lanka	23,229,470	-	South Asia
41	**Syria**	**25,620,427**	1	**Western Asia**
42	Tajikistan	10,786,734	-	Central Asia
43	**Thailand**	**71,619,863**	5	**Southeast Asia**
44	Timor–Leste	1,418,517	-	Southeast Asia
45	**Turkey**	**87,685,426**	3	**Western Asia**
46	Turkmenistan	7,618,847	-	Central Asia
47	United Arab Emirates	11,346,000	-	Western Asia
48	Uzbekistan	37,053,428	-	Central Asia
49	Vietnam	101,598,527	-	Southeast Asia
50	Yemen	41,773,878	-	Western Asia
	Taiwan *	**23,073,123**	1	**East Asia**
Selected	17 *	1,253,753,247	31	7 W; 5SE; 3S; 3E

The regional classifications which were used in this paper were taken from [12] https://unstats.un.org/unsd/methodology/m49/ (accessed on 4 July 2025)]: *East Asia*: China, China Macao, China Hong Kong, Japan, Mongolia, North Korea, Korea. *Southeast Asia:* Brunei, Cambodia, Indonesia, Laos, Malaysia, Myanmar, Philippines, Singapore, Thailand, Timor–Leste, Vietnam. *South Asia*: Afghanistan, Bangladesh, Bhutan, India, Iran, Maldives, Nepal, Pakistan, Sri Lanka. *Western Asia:* Armenia, Azerbaijan, Bahrain, Cyprus, Georgia, Iraq, Israel, Jordan, Kuwait, Lebanon, Oman, Palestine, Qatar, Saudi Arabia, Syria, Turkey, United Arab Emirates, Yemen. *Central Asia:* Kazakhstan, Kyrgyzstan, Tajikistan, Turkmenistan, Uzbekistan. (* Taiwan is not included in 50 by [12]). We selected 31 papers from 18 states (in bold in Table A1), focusing our investigation on approximately 65% (≈1,253,753,247) of the total Asian population without China and India (≈1,924,127,566).

References

1. Yoshinaga-Itano, C. Benefits of early intervention for Children with Hearing Loss. *Otolaryngol. Clin. N. Am.* **1999**, *32*, 1089–1102. [CrossRef]

2. Downs, M.P.; Yoshinaga-Itano, C. The Efficacy of early identification and intervention in children with hearing impairment. *Pediatr. Clin. N. Am.* **1999**, *46*, 79–87. [CrossRef]
3. Kemp, D.T. Stimulated acoustic emissions from within the human auditory system. *J. Acoust. Soc. Am.* **1978**, *64*, 1386–1391. [CrossRef] [PubMed]
4. Mason, J.A.; Hermann, K.R. Universal infant hearing screening by automated auditory brainstem response measurement. *Pediatrics* **1998**, *101*, 221–228. [CrossRef]
5. Edmond, K.; Chadha, S.; Hunnicutt, C.; Strobel, N.; Manchaiah, V.; Yoshinga-Itano, C.; Universal Newborn Hearing Screening (UNHS) Review Group. Effectiveness of universal newborn hearing screening: A systematic review and meta-analysis. *J. Glob. Health* **2022**, *12*, 12006. [CrossRef]
6. Zimatore, G.; Fetoni, A.R.; Paludetti, G.; Cavagnaro, M.; Podda, M.V.; Troiani, D. Post-processing analysis of transient-evoked otoacoustic emissions to detect 4 kHz-notch hearing impairment—A pilot study. *Med. Sci. Monit.* **2011**, *17*, MT41–MT49. [CrossRef]
7. Probst, R.; Lonsbury-Martin, B.L.; Martin, G.K. A review of otoacoustic emissions. *J. Acoust. Soc. Am.* **1991**, *89*, 2027–2067. [CrossRef] [PubMed]
8. Hatzopoulos, S.; Cardinali, L.; Skarżyński, P.H.; Zimatore, G. The Otoacoustic Emissions in the Universal Neonatal Hearing Screening: An Update on the European Data (2004 to 2024). *Children* **2024**, *11*, 1276. [CrossRef]
9. Hatzopoulos, S.; Cardinali, L.; Skarzynski, P.H.; Zimatore, G. The Otoacoustic Emissions in the Universal Neonatal Hearing Screening: A Scoping Review Update on the African Data (2004 to 2024). *Children* **2025**, *12*, 141. [CrossRef]
10. Hatzopoulos, S.; Cardinali, L.; Skarzynski, P.H.; Adewunmi, A.T.; Zimatore, G. Early Hearing Interventions for Children with Hearing Loss in Africa: A 21-Year Scoping Review (2004–2025). *Children* **2025**, *12*, 864. [CrossRef] [PubMed]
11. Neumann, K.; Euler, H.A.; Chadha, S.; White, K.R. A Survey on the Global Status of Newborn and Infant Hearing Screening. *J. Early Hear. Detect. Interv.* **2020**, *2*, 63–84. [CrossRef]
12. Worlmeter Website. Available online: https://www.worldometers.info/world-population/asia-population/ (accessed on 4 July 2025).
13. Falerina, R.; Nugroho, P.S.; Purnami, N.; Salsabila, F.A. A Comparison of Otoacoustic Emissions Examination Results as Early Hearing Screening in Normal and Infants at Risk of Hearing Loss. *Bali Med. J.* **2023**, *12*, 1640–1644. [CrossRef]
14. Saki, N.; Bayat, A.; Hoseinabadi, R.; Nikakhlagh, S.; Karimi, M.; Dashti, R. Universal Newborn Hearing Screening in Southwestern Iran. *Int. J. Pediatr. Otorhinolaryngol.* **2017**, *97*, 89–92. [CrossRef]
15. Gilbey, P.; Kraus, C.; Ghanayim, R.; Sharabi-Nov, A.; Bretler, S. Universal Newborn Hearing Screening in Zefat, Israel: The First Two Years. *Int. J. Pediatr. Otorhinolaryngol.* **2013**, *77*, 97–100. [CrossRef] [PubMed]
16. Ziv, O.; Danovitch, M.; Kaplan, D.M.; Tailakh, M.A.; Gorali, R.; Kurtzman, L.; Kordeluk, S.; El-Saied, S.; Slovik, Y.; Cohen, O. Cochlear Implantation Compliance among Minorities at High Risk for Hearing Impairment Following Universal Newborn Hearing Screening. *Eur. Arch. Otorhinolaryngol.* **2024**, *281*, 2877–2882. [CrossRef]
17. Farladansky-Gershnabel, S.; Kariv, L.; Schreiber, H.; Ravid, D.; Cohen, G.; Biron-Shental, T.; Kovo, M.; Krivoshey, R.E.; Arnon, S. Targeting Risk Factors for False-Positive Outcomes in Newborn Hearing Screening: A Focus on Mode of Delivery—A Case-Control Study. *Eur. Arch. Otorhinolaryngol.* 2025. *online ahead of print*. [CrossRef] [PubMed]
18. Fukushima, K.; Mimaki, N.; Fukuda, S.; Nishizaki, K. Pilot Study of Universal Newborn Hearing Screening in Japan: District-Based Screening Program in Okayama. *Ann. Otol. Rhinol. Laryngol.* **2008**, *117*, 166–171. [CrossRef]
19. Sato, T.; Nakazawa, M.; Takahashi, S.; Mizuno, T.; Ishikawa, K.; Yamada, T. Outcomes of regional-based newborn hearing screening for 35,461 newnorns for 5 years in Akita, Japan. *J. Pediatr. Otorhinolaryngol.* **2020**, *131*, 109870. [CrossRef]
20. Qanawati, L.; Alasir, R.; Gammoh, Y.; Marzouqah, R. The Association between Marriage Consanguinity and Hearing Loss in Jordan: A Retrospective Analysis. *Univ. J. Public Health* **2024**, *12*, 307–314. [CrossRef]
21. Abdullah, A.; Dahari, K.; Tamil, A.; Rohana, J.; Razif, M.; Shareena, I. The Prevalence of Hearing Loss Among Babies in the Neonatal Intensive Care Unit in a Tertiary Hospital in Malaysia. *Medeni. Med. J.* **2020**, *35*, 116–120. [CrossRef]
22. Wong, Y.; Mazlan, R.; Wahab, N.; Ja'afar, R.; Bani, N.; Abdullah, N. Quality Measures of a Multicentre Universal Newborn Hearing Screening Program in Malaysia. *J. Med.* **2021**, *28*, 238–242. [CrossRef]
23. Shrestha, B.L.; Karmacharya, S.; Dhakal, A.; Kc, A.K.; Shrestha, K.S.; Pradhan, A.; Rajbhandari, P.; Pokharel, M. Universal Neonatal Hearing Screening: An Experience at a Tertiary Care Hospital. *Kathmandu Univ. Med. J.* **2020**, *18*, 160–164. [CrossRef] [PubMed]
24. Kolethekkata, A.; Abria, R.; Hlaiwaha, O.; Harasib, Z.; Omrani, C.A.; Sulaiman, C.A.A.; Bahlani, D.H.; Jaradi, M.A.; Mathew, J. Limitations and Drawbacks of the Hospital-Based Universal Neonatal Hearing Screening Program: First Report from the Arabian Peninsula and Insights. *Int. J. Pediatr. Otorhinolaryngol.* **2020**, *132*, 109926. [CrossRef]
25. Pyarali, M.; Akhtar, S.; Adeel, M.; Mallick, S.A.; Uneeb, S.N.; Aslam, A. Neonatal Hearing Screening Programme and Challenges Faced by the Developing Country: A Tertiary Care Hospital Experience. *J. Pak. Med. Assoc.* **2023**, *73*, 1788–1793. [CrossRef]

https://doi.org/10.3390/children13010060

26. Labra, P.J.P.; Mejia, O.A.D.; Ricalde, R.R.; Catangay-Ombao, J.V.; Dela Cruz, A.P.C.; Ambrocio, G.M.C.; Capistrano, M.G.; Eugenio, N.O. Implementation of Universal Newborn Hearing Screening in the Philippines: A Survey of Registered Newborn Hearing Centers. *Acta Med. Philipp.* **2023**, *57*, 15–20. [CrossRef]
27. Habib, H.S.; Abdelgaffar, H. Neonatal Hearing Screening with Transient Evoked Otoacoustic Emissions in Western Saudi Arabia. *Int. J. Pediatr. Otorhinolaryngol.* **2005**, *69*, 839–842. [CrossRef]
28. Alanazi, A.A. Referral and lost to system rates of two newborn hearing screening programs in Saudi Arabia. *Int. J. Neonatal. Screen.* **2020**, *6*, 50. [CrossRef]
29. Elbeltagy, R.; AlObayed, W.; Mashbri, S.; Alrasheed, R.; Albakiri, R.; Almulayfi, M.; Alkahtani, R. Delayed-Onset Hearing Loss in First-Grade Students Who Previously Passed the Newborn Hearing Screening. *Front. Pediatr.* **2025**, *13*, 1623225. [CrossRef] [PubMed]
30. Jayagobi, P.A.; Yeoh, A.; Hee, K.Y.; Lim, L.S.B.; Choo, K.P.; Kun Kiaang, H.T.; Daniel, L.M. Hearing Screening Outcome in Neonatal Intensive Care Unit Graduates from a Tertiary Care Centre in Singapore. *Child. Care Health Dev.* **2020**, *46*, 104–110. [CrossRef] [PubMed]
31. Tang, J.Z.; Ng, P.G.; Loo, J.H. Do All Infants with Congenital Hearing Loss Meet the 1-3-6 Criteria? A Study of a 10-Year Cohort from a Universal Newborn Hearing Screening Programme in Singapore. *Int. J. Audiol.* **2023**, *62*, 795–804. [CrossRef] [PubMed]
32. Kim, B.G.; Shin, J.W.; Park, H.J.; Kim, J.M.; Kim, U.K.; Choi, J.Y. Limitations of Hearing Screening in Newborns with PDS Mutations. *Int. J. Pediatr. Otorhinolaryngol.* **2013**, *77*, 833–837. [CrossRef] [PubMed]
33. Lee, J.M.; Lee, H.J.; Jung, J.; Moon, I.S.; Kim, S.H.; Kim, J.; Choi, J.Y. Lessons from an Analysis of Newborn Hearing Screening Data for Children with Cochlear Implants. *Otol. Neurotol.* **2019**, *40*, e909–e917. [CrossRef] [PubMed]
34. Kaplama, M.E.; Yukkaldiran, A.; Ak, S. Newborn hearing screening results: Comparison of Syrian and Turkish newborns; factors influencing the difference. *J. Pediatr. Otorhinolaryngol.* **2020**, *138*, 110390. [CrossRef]
35. Wu, C.C.; Hung, C.C.; Lin, S.Y.; Hsieh, W.S.; Tsao, P.N.; Lee, C.N.; Su, Y.N.; Hsu, C.J. Newborn Genetic Screening for Hearing Impairment: A Preliminary Study at a Tertiary Center. *PLoS ONE* **2011**, *6*, e22314. [CrossRef] [PubMed]
36. Srisuparp, P.; Gleebbur, R.; Ngerncham, S.; Chonpracha, J.; Singkampong, J. High-Risk Neonatal Hearing Screening Program Using Automated Screening Device Performed by Trained Nursing Personnel at Siriraj Hospital: Yield and Feasibility. *J. Med. Assoc. Thai.* **2005**, *88*, S176–S182. [PubMed]
37. Poonual, W.; Navacharoen, N.; Kangsanarak, J.; Namwongprom, S. Risk Factors for Hearing Loss in Infants under Universal Hearing Screening Program in Northern Thailand. *J. Multidiscip. Healthc.* **2015**, *9*, 1–5. [CrossRef]
38. Poonual, W.; Navacharoen, N.; Kangsanarak, J.; Namwongprom, S. Outcome of Early Identification and Intervention on Infants with Hearing Loss under Universal Hearing Screening Program. *J. Med. Assoc. Thai.* **2017**, *100*, 197–206. [PubMed]
39. Poonual, W.; Navacharoen, N.; Kangsanarak, J.; Namwongprom, S.; Saokaew, S. Hearing Loss Screening Tool (COBRA Score) for Newborns in Primary Care Setting. *Korean J. Pediatr.* **2017**, *60*, 353–358. [CrossRef]
40. Pitathawatchai, P.; Khaimook, W.; Kirtsreesakul, V. Pilot implementation of newborn hearing screening programme at four hospitals in southern Thailand. *Bull. World Health Organ.* **2019**, *97*, 663–671. [CrossRef]
41. Tatli, M.M.; Serbetcioglu, M.B.; Duman, N.; Kumral, A.; Kirkim, G.; Ogun, B.; Ozkan, H. Feasibility of Neonatal Hearing Screening Program with Two-Stage Transient Otoacoustic Emissions in Turkey. *Pediatr. Int.* **2007**, *49*, 161–166. [CrossRef]
42. Tasci, Y.; Muderris, I.I.; Erkaya, S.; Altinbas, S.; Yucel, H.; Haberal, A. Newborn Hearing Screening Programme Outcomes in a Research Hospital from Turkey. *Child. Care Health Dev.* **2010**, *36*, 317–322. [CrossRef]
43. Yılmazer, R.; Yazıcı, M.Z.; Erdim, İ.; Kaya, H.K.; Özcan Dalbudak, Ş.; Kayhan, T.F. Follow-Up Results of Newborns after Hearing Screening at a Training and Research Hospital in Turkey. *J. Int. Adv. Otol.* **2016**, *12*, 55–60. [CrossRef] [PubMed]
44. Zizlavsky, S.; Supartono, N.; Zachreini, I.; Bashiruddin, J.; Haryuna, T.S.H.; Savitri, E.; Mayangsari, I.D.; Tamin, S.; Priyono, H.; Ranakusuma, R.W.; et al. Factors associated with time of diagnosis and habilitation of congenital hearing loss in Indonesia: A multicenter study. *Int. J. Ped. Otorhinolaryngol.* **2022**, *163*, 111369. [CrossRef] [PubMed]
45. Joint Committee on Infant Hearing. Year 2007 position statement: Principles and guidelines for early hearing detection and intervention programs. *Pediatrics* **2007**, *120*, 898–921. [CrossRef] [PubMed]
46. Page, M.J.; McKenzie, J.E.; Bossuyt, P.M.; Boutron, I.; Hoffmann, T.C.; Mulrow, C.D.; Shamseer, L.; Tetzlaff, J.M.; Akl, E.A.; Brennan, S.E.; et al. The PRISMA 2020 statement: An updated guideline for reporting systematic reviews. *BMJ* **2021**, *372*, n71. [CrossRef]

https://doi.org/10.3390/children13010060

children

MDPI

Review

Early Hearing Interventions for Children with Hearing Loss in Africa: A 21-Year Scoping Review (2004–2025)

Stavros Hatzopoulos [1], Ludovica Cardinali [2], Piotr Henryk Skarzynski [3,4,5], Abiodun T. Adewunmi [6] and Giovanna Zimatore [7,*]

1 Clinic of Audiology & ENT, University of Ferrara, 44121 Ferrara, Italy; sdh1@unife.it
2 Department of Life Science, Health, and Health Professions, Link Campus University, 00165 Rome, Italy; l.cardinali@unilink.it
3 Heart Failure and Cardiac Rehabilitation Department, Faculty of Medicine and Dentistry, Medical University of Warsaw, 02-005 Warsaw, Poland; piotrhskarzynski@gmail.com
4 Institute of Sensory Organs, 05-830 Nadarzyn, Poland
5 World Hearing Center, Department of Teleaudiology and Screening, Institute of Physiology and Pathology of Hearing, 02-042 Warsaw, Poland
6 Department of Special Education, University of Ibadan, Ibadan 200005, Nigeria; habins.city@gmail.com
7 Department of Theoretical and Applied Sciences Applied Physics, Campus University, 22060 Novedrate, Italy
* Correspondence: giovanna.zimatore@uniecampus.it

Abstract: Background: The objectives of this scoping review were (a) to identify the most recent (in a 21-year span) literature information about hearing intervention programs in Africa and (b) to provide data on the intervention practices, policies and the factors prohibiting the larger diffusion of the hearing technologies in the African states. Methods: Queries were conducted via the PubMed and Scopus databases for the time window from 2005 to 2025. The mesh terms used were "hearing aids", "cochlear implants", and "hearing intervention Africa". Only research articles and review papers were considered as good candidates. The standard English language filter was not used, so as to also identify information from non-English-speaking scientific communities and groups. Results: Data from eight papers were considered, reflecting the hearing intervention practices of six African states. These reports, although integral in themselves, examine different aspects of children's hearing identification and grouping the information was not entirely feasible. It is assumed that since there are no organized or centralized NHS programs in the African states, the primary driver of hearing identification appears to be parental vigilance. The cochlear implant intervention is not very diffused mainly due to complex economic factors of the weak African economies. Anecdotal data refer to cultural bias versus hearing intervention technology, but this information needs further elucidation. Conclusions: The information on the African programs on hearing intervention policies is quite scarce, as in the case of African NHS. Within this context, it is very important to convince audiologists and ENTs from the African localized programs to publish their data in mainstream channels so that new information can be assessed.

Keywords: hearing aids; cochlear implants; early hearing intervention; Africa

1. Introduction

Childhood hearing loss constitutes a considerable public health issue, particularly in countries with low or middle incomes where access to early diagnostic and intervention services is restricted [1]. Early hearing detection and intervention (EHDI) programs, which include universal neonatal hearing screening (UNHS), timely hearing aid (HA) fitting, and cochlear implants (CIs), are essential to mitigate the impact of congenital hearing loss on speech, cognitive, and social development. In high-income countries, the systematic implementation of UNHS protocols has enabled the early identification of hearing impairment, facilitating prompt auditory intervention during critical periods of neuroplasticity. Early auditory access through hearing devices, coupled with consistent use, has been shown to significantly improve linguistic and developmental outcomes in affected children [2]. The earlier-implanted children are more proficient than later-implanted children in their phonological development [3,4]. Despite the established benefits, the implementation of UNHS and subsequent rehabilitative interventions across the African continent remains inconsistent and fragmented, with substantial disparities in program coverage, accessibility, and follow-up services.

A recent review [5] highlighted the severe lack of comprehensive NHS programs across the African continent, with available data reflecting localized initiatives in only a handful of countries and often limited to urban centers. Despite efforts to screen neonates using otoacoustic emissions (OAEs) and automated auditory brainstem response (AABR) technologies, the review underscored significant gaps in follow-up care, intervention strategies, and published outcomes, particularly regarding the use of devices such as HAs and CIs for children identified with hearing loss. Moreover, high loss-to-follow-up rates and infrastructural challenges, such as the shortage of trained audiologists and the social stigma associated with deafness, further compromise the effectiveness of these programs.

Given the critical role of early auditory intervention in improving developmental routes for children with hearing loss, it is essential to assess the extent to which HAs and CIs have been utilized among the African pediatric population over the past two decades. This scoping review complements the NHS and EHDI African data we have previously presented and focuses on the next step after the NHS, that is, on the hearing intervention practices available to the African children. The purpose of this work is to provide possible guidance for expanding access to effective auditory rehabilitation across the continent by identifying achievements, barriers, and gaps.

2. Materials and Methods

In various contexts, Africa is divided into the northern region and the sub-Saharan region, which includes 54 states. In this review, we considered the whole continent without any specific geographical divisions. As in the previous review analysis of the African neonatal hearing screening data, we have focused our investigation on the 84.45% of the total African population (1,532,073,577) that was measured in 2024 and reported in terms of the 25 most population-dense African states.

Since the present manuscript is the continuation of the paper on the African NHS and EDHI practices [5], we initially chose a 20-year window (2004–2024) to search for information. Due to the small manuscript yield of the initial searches, the year 2025 was added to the search window, which was conducted in April 2025 and followed the PRISMA 2020 guidelines. (See PRISMA Checklist Supplementary Materials Table S1). The queries utilized the following three keywords and phrases (mesh terms): "hearing aids", "cochlear implants", and "hearing intervention Africa". The PubMed and Scopus databases were assessed, and research articles and review papers were considered as good candidates. One case report was also included due to the scarcity of information on the type of CIs used in the intervention practices. The review papers included in the study were assessed and controlled for possible overlap of information with the accepted research papers. The standard English language filter was not used, so as to identify possible information from non-English-speaking (i.e., French) scientific communities and groups. Papers related to hearing interventions outside the African continent were not considered. The inclusion and exclusion criteria are reported in Table 1.

Table 1. Selection criteria.

Inclusion Criteria
• Article type: research, review papers, and eligible case reports • Article scope: article reports on hearing intervention practices—including hearing aids and cochlear implants—among African children • Participants: children (<18 y) • Area of application: articles that conducted research in the field of deaf mitigation by HAs and CIs • Language: English, French • Publication period: last 21 years (considering only 3 months of 2025)
Exclusion Criteria
• Article type: opinions, commentaries, letters to the editor, or conference papers • Article scope: not related to HAs and CIs • Participants: animals, adults • Area of application: not related to hearing intervention practices (classified as "wrong outcome"), hearing interventions outside the African territory • Language: none • Publication period: published >21 years ago

Two independent reviewers reviewed the available material (38 manuscripts) and distilled the final number of eligible papers to 8. The quality criteria for the manuscript selection included: (i) the publication being in a peer-reviewed journal and (ii) the candidate paper clearly showing a scientific methodology style.

It should be noted that we were able to additionally identify (through the reference sections of the accepted manuscripts) a number of additional articles. These were published in African journals such as the *Pan African Medical Journal* and the *South Sudan Medical Journal*, which are not indexed in PubMed or Scopus. These papers were excluded from the submission evaluation filtering procedure. Theoretically, these sources (lacking an impact factor) would undermine the quality standards we have established for this scoping review, but considering the extreme lack of information, the presented data are reported in Appendix A and should be treated as anecdotal additional.

In Figure 1, the PRISMA flowchart process is reported. The candidate papers for this review are reported in Table 2.

Table 2. The 8 eligible papers after the filtering process: The national data are presented in alphabetical order.

n	Country	Type of Hearing Impairment	Sample Size (*n*)	Period of Data Collection	Type of Paper	Author (First)	Publication Year
1	Egypt	Bilateral prelingual severe to profound SHL	90	July 2015–January 2017	Validation study (cross-sectional cohort)	El-Dessouky [6]	2019
2	Malawi	Severe to profound SHL	19	2014–2022	Case series study	Mulwafu [7]	2025
3	Nigeria	Congenital and early-onset childhood HL	223	January 2008–December 2013	Retrospective descriptive study	Adedeji [1]	2015
4	South Africa	Congenital and progressive HL	45	2004 (retrospective)	Cross-sectional quantitative survey	Jessop [8]	2007
5	South Africa	Severe to profound SHL	7	2022–2023	Qualitative exploratory study (mothers interviewed)	Kanji [9]	2024

Table 2. *Cont.*

n	Country	Type of Hearing Impairment	Sample Size (*n*)	Period of Data Collection	Type of Paper	Author (First)	Publication Year
6	South Africa	Bilateral profound SHL with cochlear malformation	1	2015	Case report	Atiya [10]	2018
7	South Africa	Not explicitly specified, focus on the family experience post-implant	19 CI	COVID-19 epidemic period, (2020–2022, not specified precisely)	Qualitative conceptual framework (by parents)	de Beer [11]	2024
8	Sub-Saharan Africa *	Severe-to-profound congenital SHL	Not specified	2012	Economic evaluation study	Emmett [12]	2015

* Kenya, Nigeria, Malawi, South Africa, Rwanda, and Uganda.

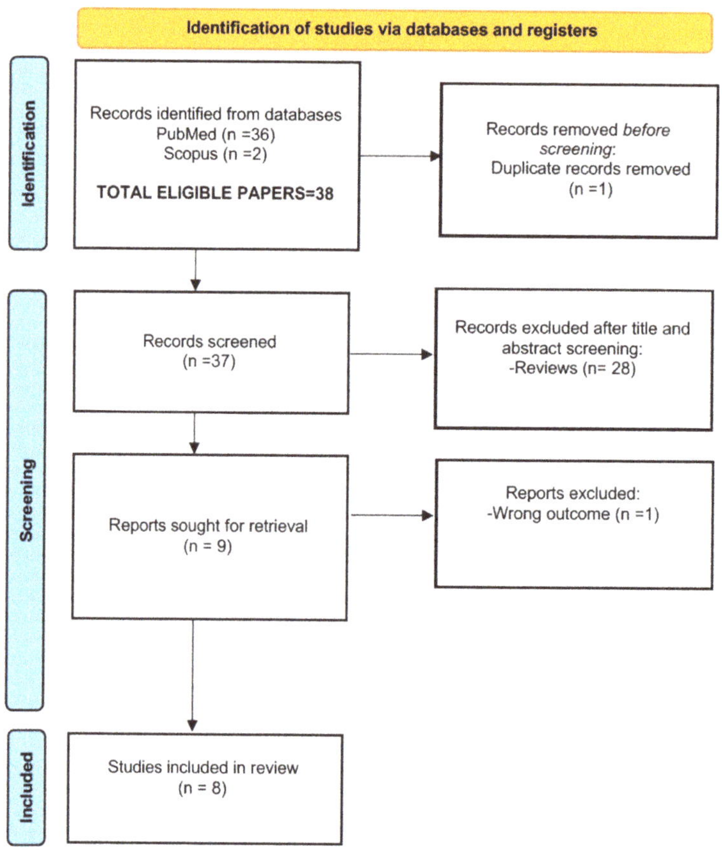

Figure 1. Flow diagram of the literature search, according to the PRISMA criteria (http://www.prisma-statement.org/, accessed 30 July 2024), with the steps followed in the manuscript selection procedure. After the application of the selection criteria, the initial 38 manuscripts were reduced to 8.

3. Results

The data were classified alphabetically according to the country of origin. Considering that there are no organized hearing screening practices or early detection and hearing intervention programs in Africa [5], it is reasonable to postulate that the hearing deficits of the assisted children are identified by members of their families. This point, however, requires further elucidation and additional research.

Three of the eight papers selected were published in the last five years. Two papers were retrospective studies, and two were qualitative studies. The papers included data from one patient (a case report) to a maximum of 223 subjects. All these studies were conducted on a limited number of implanted subjects, except for one involving both CIs and HAs. Of the eight papers (for a total of 404 subjects), four reported data from severe SHL cases.

Table 3 synthesizes key themes across studies, noting both empirical results and modeled data.

Table 3. The 8 eligible papers after the filtering process: a comparative summary of key data points.

n	Study	Country	Age at Implantation	Post-Implantation Outcomes	Hearing Device Usage
1	El-Dessouky et al. (2019) [6]	Egypt	Mean: ~3 years	Improved auditory skills on the Egyptian Arabic scale	Consistent CI use with structured benefit
2	Mulwafu et al. (2025) [7]	Malawi	Median: ~4.8 years	Positive audiometric and speech perception results	CI was used consistently in a clinical setting
3	Adedeji et al. (2015) [1]	Nigeria	Not specified precisely; often delayed	Limited data; outcomes impacted by late diagnosis	Limited access and affordability issues
4	Jessop et al. (2007) [8]	South Africa	Range: 1–10 years	Parents report developmental progress	Regular CI use; variable based on support
5	Kanji et al. (2024) [9]	South Africa	Range: 2–6 years; delays are common	Emotional and social challenges highlighted	Use influenced by therapy access
6	Atiya et al. (2018) [10]	South Africa	12 months	Success with a hybrid device in partial hearing preservation	Consistent use of CI
7	de Beer et al. (2024) [11]	South Africa	Varies; includes early and late	High family impact; importance of support	Regular use tied to family support
8	Emmett et al. (2015) [12]	Sub-Saharan Africa *	Modeled early vs. late	CI is cost-effective in early implantation scenarios	Modeled consistent CI use

* Kenya, Nigeria, Malawi, South Africa, Rwanda, Uganda.

Analytically, the reported intervention policies are listed below, by African state, in alphabetical order.

3.1. Egypt

El-Dessouky et al. (2019) [6] conducted a validation study of the Arabic version of the auditory skills checklist using a cohort of 90 Egyptian children (mean age 36–72 months) with bilateral severe-to-profound prelingual hearing loss (since birth), all fitted with CIs. The children had no experience with CIs, but they were previously fitted with hearing aids. The paper offers no information on the time of HA fitting. The study reinforced the utility of culturally and linguistically adapted assessment tools in tracking auditory development. The cohort benefited from structured intervention and follow-up protocols, demonstrating significant post-implant auditory skills development within a 3-year period. Detailed scores of linguistic development were reported in terms of detection, identification, short-term auditory memory, supra-segmental discrimination, segmental discrimination, and linguistic auditory processing.

3.2. Malawi

Data from the state of Malawi are available from Mulwafu et al. (2025) [7], detailing the early outcomes from the country's first cochlear implantation program. This paper presents the most detailed information about the linguistic evaluation of the implanted children. The paper reports data from 17 patients who received a CI from 2014 to 2022. The subjects presented postlingual HL and received the Synchrony FLEX 28 implant from Medel. Deafness was identified at 8.7 ± 6.3 y and the implantation was conducted at 10.8 ± 4.7 y. Audiometric and speech perception improvements were observed, demonstrating promising clinical results despite infrastructural limitations. The most significant results were obtained in the Monosyllabic Tronchee Polysyllabic test (MTP), where the authors declared: "14 children (82.3%) achieved scores of 20 or more out of the maximum 24. The remaining 3 children achieved scores of 12, 2, and 1. In the MTP syllables test, 12 children (70.5%) achieved scores of 20 or more out of 24. The remaining 5 children achieved scores of 18, 18, 17, 7, and 1."

3.3. Nigeria

In Nigeria, a retrospective descriptive study conducted by Adedeji et al. (2015) [1] reviewed 223 children with congenital and early-onset childhood hearing loss. The study highlighted significant delays (not defined in the paper) in diagnosis and intervention, largely due to limited audiological services and public awareness. The primary interventions reported included HAs and CIs, though access remained restricted to urban tertiary facilities. This underscores the need for community-based screening and early intervention programs.

Due to the scarcity of the reported material, we are presenting in Appendix A additional from one of the authors (A.A.). The data were derived from a Government Northern Central Hospital in Nigeria, and show a constant flat rate of HA requests from 2021. Data on CIs are also presented. It should be noted that the northern part of Nigeria consists of more Hausas who hold the belief that whatever happens to people is from God, which may reduce their motivation to actively pursue hearing interventions such as acquiring HA, as well as other health-related treatments. These anecdotal conclusions still need validation through questionnaires or other means.

3.4. South Africa

South Africa had the most extensive coverage across the literature, regarding data on HAs and CIs, spanning 17 years and represented by four articles. According to Emmett et al. [12], South Africa is currently the only country within the low/middle-income context of sub-Saharan Africa that has established a national CI program.

Jessop et al. [8] described 45 cases from the Pretoria CI program. Their paper was based on questionnaire data from queries sent to 71 families, of which only 45 were returned. The age of implantation was varied from 12 months to 10 years. The main aim of the paper was to describe the CI outcomes, as perceived by their parents. The reported causes of hearing loss, in declining order, were unknown, meningitis, genetic syndrome, prenatal complications, birth trauma, rubella, and cytomegalovirus. In terms of linguistic development, the authors declared, "More children in this study were using single words than more complex word combinations, however, an even larger group was using mature sentence forms. This indicated that in the present cross-sectional study, more children were in either the earlier, or the more advanced stages of language acquisition than in the middle stages".

In Soweto, South Africa, a CI program was developed at the Chris Hani Baragwanath Academic Hospital. This is one of the few fully state-funded programs in the country and targets a poor population [10]. The paper provides data from a single CI case, using Cochlea's Hybrid CI24REH device on a male subject 12 months old. In terms of linguistic development, the authors reported that, according to the results of the 34-month-old Rossetti Infant–Toddler Language Scale, language expression was measured at 15 months and understanding at 12 months. The subject scored between 30 and 33 months on both language expression and understanding when it was repeated at 44 months, indicating that his language delay had considerably decreased during the preceding 12 months.

De Beer et al. [11] explored family perspectives post-implantation, emphasizing the social and emotional dimensions of intervention in a sample of 29 parents of 26 pediatric CI recipients (younger than 18 years) who had been implanted for at least 12 months at the time of data collection. Concept maps were derived in order to weigh the impact of various factors on the life of the implanted subjects and according to the authors "The maps revealed six important areas of social impact, namely (i) Financial Outlay and Supports; (ii) Education and Therapy; (iii) Responsibilities and Sacrifices; (iv) Extended Family and Community; (v) Spouses and Siblings and (vi) Achievements and Enrichments."

Lastly, Kanji et al. [9] conducted qualitative interviews with parents of children who received CIs, stressing the challenges related to costs and post-operative support.

Collectively, the South African studies document a structured, albeit resource-limited, cochlear implantation infrastructure, with growing attention to holistic, family-centered care.

3.5. Sub-Saharan Area (Kenya, Malawi, Rwanda, and Uganda)

These countries were primarily examined in a cost-effectiveness analysis by Emmett et al. [12], comparing the implementation of CIs and deaf education. While specific sample sizes per country were not disaggregated, the study supported the feasibility and value of cochlear implantation within these low-resource settings when paired with sustained rehabilitation and education. The interesting part of the study was that local reference clinicians (who were also co-authors) collected national data regarding CIs, but the analytical information is not available in the paper.

The authors reached interesting and optimistic conclusions: (i) South Africa has the most developed socioeconomic structure in the sub-Saharan group, which makes cochlear implantation extremely cost-effective; (ii) Nigeria shows that CIs can reach the cost-effective threshold and in order to reach 30% of the estimated children in need, the current Nigerian implant program, which only provides five implants annually, must increase by more than 500%; (3) the other countries in the study show the potential to extend their CI programs to rural areas that have not historically had access to this technology. To create strong national CI initiatives, philanthropic, academic, and commercial partnerships are required in Kenya, Rwanda, Uganda, and Malawi. In these growing economies, device cost and related maintenance have a significant impact.

4. Discussion

The aim of the paper was to collect as much information as possible on the reported hearing intervention policies in the African states. Due to the lack of organized neonatal hearing programs and other relevant information, the data of this review refer to intervention practices and not intervention policies and strategies. The data collected show a significant scarcity of information, in terms of the selected practices, the intervention timing, intervention complications, etc. In order to elucidate better this aspect, we present in Figure 2 geographical data regarding the status of African hearing screening and hearing interventions: (i) the top map presents the African states who have reported neonatal hearing screening (NHS) practices (data from a previous review paper by [5]), and (ii) the bottom map shows the African states offering hearing intervention programs: Egypt,

Kenya, Malawi, Nigeria, Rwanda, South Africa, and Uganda. All active programs are shown in green color.

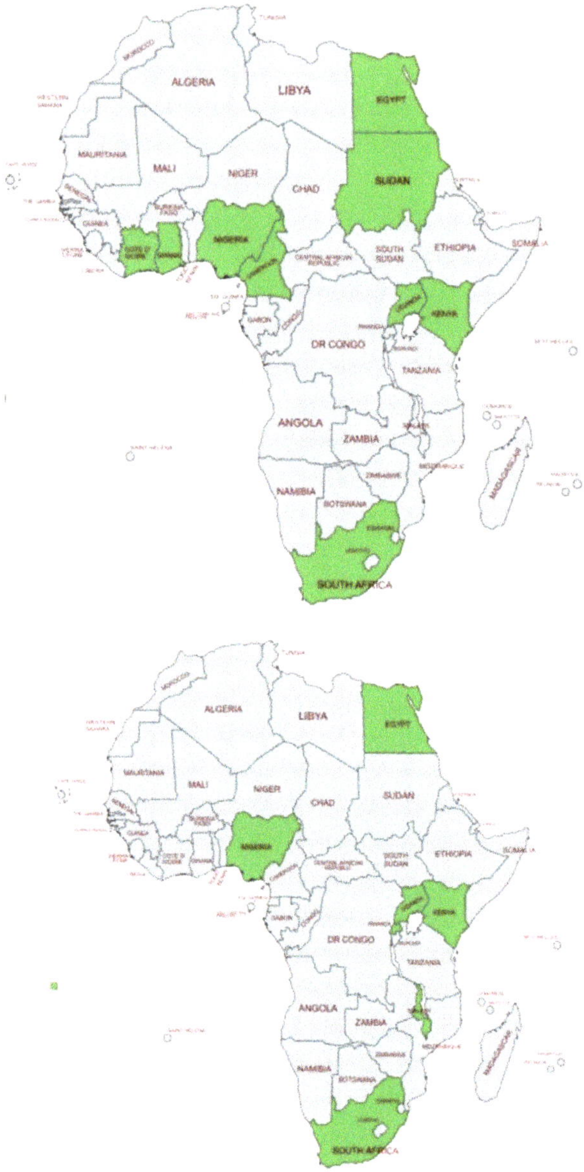

Figure 2. Comparison of the African states reporting newborn hearing screening (top) and those reporting hearing intervention policies (bottom). Countries with active hearing programs or hearing intervention activities are shown in green. The map at the top shows the countries where hearing screening data are reported in the literature [5]. The map at the bottom shows the countries where information on hearing intervention policies is reported, including Egypt, Kenya, Malawi, Nigeria, Rwanda, South Africa, and Uganda.

This figure is designed to illustrate the lack of overlap between early hearing detection efforts and actual hearing intervention practices. Notably, regions with reported hearing screening activities are often the same regions where interventions such as HAs and CIs are implemented, suggesting that without early identification of hearing loss, further intervention is unlikely to occur. Otherwise, the fact that the data from the two maps do not overlap well suggests that some partial intervention exists, even without any hearing screening basis. Based on the articles we have found in non-mainstream impact factor journals, we postulate that data on the clinical practices in the areas of hearing screening and intervention are not reported in these channels, and they are not easily traceable.

To better clarify this aspect, we show in Appendix A clinical data on HAs and CIs, which are not reported in the standard PubMed and Scopus databases. This pattern is not unexpected, as many clinical settings generate data that remain unpublished in high-impact journals—potentially due to the economic constraints of open access publishing—or are instead disseminated through non-indexed local publications. Similar underreporting has been documented in other regions globally, including within European countries, where published data on hearing screening remain limited, as highlighted in a recent study by our group [13].

The totality of collected information about the hearing intervention practices in the African states cannot be aggregated in meaningful groups, as it is quite sporadic. Unfortunately, the collected information does not allow (i) a comparison of results between the various African states, (ii) the identification of trends in government intervention policies, or (iii) the identification of the missing features in the intervention programs. Therefore, the reported outcomes are difficult to compare with the data from interventions in other parts of the world.

Nevertheless, several aspects of the hearing intervention policies can be minimally discussed, as follows.

4.1. Intervention Times

Since there are no organized hearing screening programs on the African continent, it has been postulated that children with hearing deficits eventually get assisted by members of their families, who probably monitor their hearing behavior. This is typical behavior in the Western world [14,15]. Since there is a lack of specific information on this issue, the postulate was based on anecdotal information from one of the co-authors (A.A.). The aspect of the intervention timing point is extremely important for any intervention strategy and therefore requires additional elucidation studies.

The majority of the available data with reference to CIs do not indicate the time when the subjects were implanted after being fitted with an HA. Data from papers presenting the actual age of the assisted patients with a CI are available from Egypt, Malawi, and South Africa. The minimum ages of the implanted subjects range from 10 months (South Africa) to 10.8 years (Malawi). The Egyptian data refer to a minimal age of 36 months, but for subjects who were already fitted with an HA. Although the Malawi estimates are derived from a starting pilot project, it must be noted that they are significantly larger than the recommended standards used in most European and American early detection and intervention programs that start an intervention at 6 months [14–16]. Anecdotal data in Appendix A suggest that in Nigeria and Tanzania, intervention policies are applied as early as 2 years.

4.2. Factors Inhibiting the Hearing Intervention Policies

In the previous review paper on African neonatal hearing screening, we identified a series of obstacles related to the distribution of the new screening technologies, primarily related to economic, cultural, and religious beliefs. The majority of the papers in this review (except the paper on the sub-Saharan countries by Emmett et al. [12]) do not mention any of those factors, but some anecdotal information is presented in Appendix A.

The costs of the CI part of the intervention policies are seen as the main factor inhibiting a wider distribution of assistance services from central to rural areas. This is a complex issue to affront in a third-world context, because, as Emmett et al. [12] show, the actual costs of a CI intervention include not only the cost of the device but also the costs related to hospitalization and post-intervention procedures.

Regarding the anecdotal resources:

(i) One of the authors of this review (A.A.), who has colleagues working in Nigerian hospitals, has provided anecdotal evidence suggesting that in northern Nigeria, religious beliefs significantly impede the diffusion of hearing intervention policies (see the Section 3.3). Since there are cultural issues related to the diffusion of the screening strategies, it can be safely assumed that the same concepts will impede the application of HAs and CIs to the general population. Nevertheless, these aspects need to be better clarified with well-defined questionnaires.

(ii) Anecdotal data from Senegal suggest that the costs of the screening procedures and the intervention devices are strongly prohibiting the diffusion of the intervention solutions to the general population. Again, these aspects need to be better clarified with well-defined questionnaires.

4.3. *Technologies Used in the Hearing Intervention*

From the eight papers included in the review, only one, referring to the Egyptian data, made a reference to HAs prior to implantation. Additional references were not reported, so the names of the devices and the relative clinical and hardware protocols are not known.

In terms of CI brands, the information was specified in only two papers: the Cochlear Hybrid CI24REH model in [10], and MEDEL SONATA TI and Advanced Bionics (HiRes 90K) in [6].

4.4. *Possible Limitations of the Study*

Since the number of papers in this review is low, the overall conclusions regarding the status of the African intervention policies might be biased and inconclusive.

Additionally, since we have found a number of publications not indexed in the PubMed or Scopus databases, it is reasonable to assume that there might be others as well, which we did not identify. These sources, although treated as anecdotal, might contain information useful in the context of this review.

5. Conclusions

Across these African nations, cochlear implantation emerged as the dominant intervention for severe-to-profound hearing loss. However, disparities persist in terms of access, infrastructure, and post-implantation support. Nigeria and Egypt report relatively higher sample sizes and infrastructure, while South Africa demonstrates multidimensional research on clinical and psychosocial outcomes. Kenya, Rwanda, Uganda, and Malawi represent emerging frontiers in cochlear health services, warranting further investment and research. A regional strategy to standardize care, expand audiology services, and integrate family-centered rehabilitation models is essential for sustainable impact. To create strong national HA and CI initiatives, philanthropic, academic, and commercial partnerships are strongly required.

Supplementary Materials: The following supporting information can be downloaded at: https://www.mdpi.com/article/10.3390/children12070864/s1, Table S1: PRISMA 2020 Checklist. Ref. [17] is cited in Supplementary Materials.

Author Contributions: Bibliographic search, S.H., G.Z. and L.C.; investigation, data curation: S.H., G.Z., L.C. and A.T.A.; writing—original draft preparation, S.H. and G.Z.; writing—review and editing, S.H., G.Z., A.T.A. and P.H.S. All authors have read and agreed to the published version of the manuscript.

Funding: This research received no external funding.

Institutional Review Board Statement: Not applicable.

Informed Consent Statement: Not applicable.

Data Availability Statement: The original contributions presented in this study are included in the article/Supplementary Material. Further inquiries can be directed to the corresponding author.

Conflicts of Interest: The authors declare no conflicts of interest.

Appendix A

Appendix A.1 Anecdotal Supplemental Information from Nigeria

One of the co-authors, A.A., reports the following unpublished HA (* as of May 2025) and CI trend data from Nigeria in a Government Central Northern Hospital. Usually, the fitting procedures are conducted in external clinics, and then the patients must come back to the hospital to undertake follow-up controls. As the data show, very few cases come back, and in this context, the information about problems related to HAs is not well defined. Since there is no state assistance for buying an HA device, the number of purchases is low (in comparison to referrals), but the data within the last 3 years show a moderate increase in purchases. Even in these cases, the follow-up rates are significantly low.

Table A1. The second column indicates the number of referrals for a hearing aid (HA), the second the number of purchased devices, and the third column the number of patients who have come back for a follow-up.

Year.	HA Referral.	Purchase.	Follow-Up
2021.	3.	-	-
2022.	19.	6.	1
2023.	13.	2.	1
2024.	19.	3.	1
2025. *	11.	11.	1

In terms of CIs performed in an external clinic in a time window of 12 years (2012–2024), 137 patients have received a single implant. The demographic characteristics of the patients were 2–3 y (26 cases), 4–6 y (37 cases), 7–10 y (14 cases), 10–13 y (8 cases), and >13 ys (52 cases). Additional information was not available.

Appendix A.2 Anecdotal Supplemental Information from Senegal

The data were presented in a paper by Lame et al. [18] in the *Pan African Medical Journal*. The paper examined the possibilities and the impediments of cochlear implantation in Senegal, the main factor being the high cost of the medical procedures offered in a non-insurance context.

The limitations regarding the application of hearing intervention policies are summarized by the authors. Senegal has a variety of diagnostic methods, such as auditory brainstem response and otoacoustic emissions; however, they are primarily located in the capital, Dakar, and are very expensive, particularly for those without health insurance. The anticipated cost of a full assessment for deafness is XOF 500,000 (EUR 765). This is equivalent to five and a half times the average monthly gross salary in Senegal. The Ministry of Economy, Planning, and Cooperation of Senegal reported that the average gross monthly pay in 2019 was XOF 89,730 (EUR 138). In most cases, employers or insurance companies can cover complementary examinations and surgery for employees and their families.

However, the patient still bears the burden of purchasing the implant, which is the costliest component. It is necessary to provide CI candidates and their families with financial support. There is a technological platform accessible for cochlear implantation. However, currently, only three places have implemented this type of intervention. There are not many speech therapists in the nation. There are currently fewer than ten of them, and they are responsible for all patients' rehabilitation across all specializations.

Appendix A.3 Anecdotal Supplemental Information from Tanzania

The data were presented in a paper by Kahinga et al. [19], in the *South Sudan Medical Journal*, from 39 patients (2–55 y with a mean age of 4.7 y), who were implanted in the Muhimbili National Hospital. The demographic characteristics of the patients were 2–3 y (24 cases), 4–5 y (13 cases), and >5 (2 cases). Interestingly, the authors refer to a case of a 55 y patient without any reason for why this case was included in the pool with the other data. The main causes of hearing loss were ototoxicity and birth asphyxia.

Thirty-seven patients presented with prelingual bilateral profound hearing loss. Due to the high costs of the CI, 37 out of the 39 patients were implanted with a single device. The support for the costs of the implants came from the Tanzanian government.

Data for post-operatory speech performance were available for only one case, who moved from 0 to 36 points on the Infant–Toddler Meaningful Auditory Integration Scale (IT-MAIS) over a period of 18 months, post-implantation.

This paper is the only one of the papers in this review that refers to CI post-operative complications. The authors declare that the described symptoms were "facial weakness, which was the commonest, followed by skin infection at the surgical site which led to extrusion of the device. Other complications such as meningitis, was not reported and this could be attributed to the provision of pneumococcal polysaccharide vaccine and Haemophilus influenzae vaccines prior surgery".

References

1. Adedeji, T.O.; Tobih, J.E.; Sogebi, O.A.; Daniel, A.D. Management challenges of congenital & early onset childhood hearing loss in a sub-Saharan African country. *Int. J. Pediatr. Otorhinolaryngol.* **2015**, *79*, 1625–1629. [CrossRef] [PubMed]
2. Moeller, M.P.; Hoover, B.; Peterson, B.; Stelmachowicz, P. Consistency of hearing aid use in infants with early-identified hearing loss. *Am. J. Audiol.* **2009**, *18*, 14–23. [CrossRef] [PubMed]
3. Peer, S. Turning up the volume on hearing loss in South Africa. *S. Afr. Med. J.* **2015**, *105*, 31–32. [CrossRef] [PubMed]
4. Quriba, A.S.; Hassan, E.M. Analysis of phonological criteria in Egyptian Arabic speaking children using cochlear implant. *Int. J. Pediatr. Otorhinolaryngol.* **2019**, *127*, 109637. [CrossRef] [PubMed]
5. Hatzopoulos, S.; Cardinali, L.; Skarzynski, P.H.; Zimatore, G. The Otoacoustic Emissions in the Universal Neonatal Hearing Screening: A Scoping Review Update on the African Data (2004 to 2024). *Children* **2025**, *12*, 141. [CrossRef] [PubMed]
6. El-Dessouky, H.M.; Aziz, A.A.; Sheikhany, A.R.; ElMeshmeshy, L.M. Validation of the Egyptian Arabic Assessment of Auditory Skills development using children with Cochlear Implants. *Int. J. Pediatr. Otorhinolaryngol.* **2019**, *122*, 52–59. [CrossRef] [PubMed]
7. Mulwafu, W.; Chabaluka, C.; Anderson, I.; Strachan, D.; Raine, C. Development of a Cochlear Implantation Program in Malawi: Audiometric and Speech Perception Results from a Series of Implantees. *Otolaryngol.-Head Neck Surg.* **2025**, *172*, 1109–1113. [CrossRef] [PubMed]
8. Jessop, M.; Kritzinger, A.; Venter, N. Parental perceptions of characteristics and outcomes of children and families in the Pretoria Cochlear Implant Programme. *S. Afr. J. Commun. Disord.* **2007**, *54*, 47–58. [CrossRef] [PubMed]
9. Kanji, A.; Mirkin, L.; Casoojee, A. Experiences of parents of children with cochlear implants in South Africa: An exploratory study. *Disabil. Rehabil.* **2024**, *46*, 5044–5051. [CrossRef] [PubMed]

10. Atiya, Y.; Ahmed, M.R.; Schlesinger-Michelow, D. Novel use of the Cochlear® Hybrid CI24REH cochlear implant. *Cochlear Implant. Int.* **2018**, *19*, 167–169. [CrossRef] [PubMed]
11. de Beer, C.; Bennett, R.J.; Eikelboom, R.H.; le Roux, T. Impact of paediatric cochlear implantation on family life: A conceptual framework informed by parents. *Disabil. Rehabil.* **2024**, *46*, 6410–6423. [CrossRef] [PubMed]
12. Emmett, S.D.; Tucci, D.L.; Smith, M.; Macharia, I.M.; Ndegwa, S.N.; Nakku, D.; Kaitesi, M.B.; Ibekwe, T.S.; Mulwafu, W.; Gong, W.; et al. GDP Matters: Cost Effectiveness of Cochlear Implantation and Deaf Education in Sub-Saharan Africa. *Otol. Neurotol.* **2015**, *36*, 1357–1365. [CrossRef] [PubMed]
13. Hatzopoulos, S.; Cardinali, L.; Skarżyński, P.H.; Zimatore, G. The Otoacoustic Emissions in the Universal Neonatal Hearing Screening: An Update on the European Data (2004 to 2024). *Children* **2024**, *11*, 1276. [CrossRef] [PubMed]
14. Yoshinaga-Itano, C. Benefits of early intervention for children with hearing loss. *Otolaryngol. Clin. N. Am.* **1999**, *32*, 1089–1102. [CrossRef] [PubMed]
15. Yoshinaga-Itano, C.; Carr, G.; Davis, A.; Ching, T.Y.C.; Chung, K.; Clark, J.; Harkus, S.; Kuan, M.L.; Garg, S.; Balen, S.A.; et al. Coalition for Global Hearing Health Hearing Care Pathways Working Group: Guidelines for Clinical Guidance for Readiness and Development of Evidence-Based Early Hearing Detection and Intervention Programs. *Ear Hear.* **2024**, *45*, 1071–1088. [CrossRef] [PubMed]
16. Downs, M.P.; Yoshinaga-Itano, C. The efficacy of early identification and intervention in children with hearing impairment. *Pediatr. Clin. N. Am.* **1999**, *46*, 79–87. [CrossRef] [PubMed]
17. Page, M.J.; McKenzie, J.E.; Bossuyt, P.M.; Boutron, I.; Hoffmann, T.C.; Mulrow, C.D.; Shamseer, L.; Tetzlaff, J.M.; Akl, E.A.; Brennan, S.E.; et al. The PRISMA 2020 statement: An updated guideline for reporting systematic reviews. *BMJ* **2021**, *372*, n71. [CrossRef] [PubMed]
18. Lame, C.A.; Sy, A.; Loum, B. Implantation cochléaire au Sénégal: Enjeux, limites et perspectives. *Pan Afr. Med. J.* **2023**, *45*, 12. [CrossRef] [PubMed]
19. Kahinga, A.A.; Abraham, Z.S.; Mawala, S.; Liyombo, E. Cochlear implantation and outcomes in a resource-limited setting: Experience from Tanzania. *S. Sudan Med. J.* **2022**, *15*, 50–53. [CrossRef]

children

MDPI

Review

Congenital Cytomegalovirus (cCMV) Infection as a Leading Cause of Pediatric Hearing Loss: Review

Amber Cradeur [1,†], Aaron Jackson [1,†], Erin Ware [2], Torrey L. Fourrier [3] and Gauri Mankekar [3,*,†]

1 School of Medicine, Louisiana State University Health Shreveport, 1501, King's Highway, Shreveport, LA 71103, USA; alc007@lsuhs.edu (A.C.); ajj001@lsuhs.edu (A.J.)
2 Library, Louisiana State University Health Shreveport, 1501, King's Highway, Shreveport, LA 71103, USA; eew001@lsuhs.edu
3 Department of Otolaryngology-Head and Neck Surgery, Louisiana State University Health Shreveport, 1501, King's Highway, Shreveport, LA 71103, USA; torrey.fourrier@lsuhs.edu
* Correspondence: gauri.mankekar@lsuhs.edu
† These authors contributed equally to this work.

Abstract: Background/Objectives: Congenital cytomegalovirus (cCMV) infection is a significant cause of pediatric hearing loss. However, the prevalence and characteristics of cCMV-related hearing loss remain unclear. **Methods**: A comprehensive search of major databases (PubMed, Scopus, and Web of Science) was conducted to identify studies and reviews published between 2000 and 2024 that investigated cCMV infection, testing for cCMV, and pediatric hearing loss. Studies were included if they reported on the prevalence, characteristics, current policies, and recommendations for universal cCMV testing in newborns. **Results**: This review highlights key issues: cCMV is a significant and treatable cause of pediatric hearing loss; most cCMV-related hearing loss cases presented with bilateral and profound hearing impairment; and cCMV testing is performed only for babies who fail newborn hearing screening. **Conclusions**: This narrative review highlights the significant association between cCMV infection and pediatric hearing loss. Currently, targeted cCMV testing is recommended for newborns who fail newborn hearing screening. Universal cCMV testing may facilitate early diagnosis and directed intervention and could be cost-effective in the long run.

Keywords: congenital cytomegalovirus; pediatric hearing loss; systematic review; meta-analysis; diagnostic accuracy

1. Introduction

Congenital cytomegalovirus (cCMV) infection is the leading non-genetic cause of hearing loss in the pediatric population worldwide. While most infected newborns are asymptomatic, a significant number will either be born with hearing loss or develop it later in life. The early initiation of antiviral therapy, such as ganciclovir or valganciclovir, has been reported to improve audiological and neurodevelopmental outcomes [1,2]. The European Congenital Infection Initiative (ECCI) consensus statement recommends starting valganciclovir as soon as possible for newborns with isolated sensorineural hearing loss (SNHL), as well as those with CNS symptoms [3]. However, this is controversial. A recent systematic review did not find an adequate benefit of valganciclovir on audiological outcomes in children with isolated hearing loss, late-onset hearing loss, or asymptomatic CMV [4].

Many states and hospital programs currently implement a targeted approach to cCMV screening, which involves further evaluation when a newborn does not pass their universal neonatal hearing screening. However, several studies criticize this screening method for its inadequacy in properly identifying all infected infants who are at risk of complications. While there has been significant advancement in the early detection of cCMV within recent years, secondary to the implementation of newborn hearing screening, there is still an opportunity to improve screening protocols and methodology. The current literature describes the present state of cCMV screening and detection, details the inadequacies, and largely supports the notion of implementing universal neonatal screening for cCMV.

To accurately capture the prevalence, clinical presentation, and current state of cCMV screening and detection, various phases and criteria were used in the literature search for this narrative review (Figure 1). The first phase of the literature review involved an extensive search of major databases (PubMed, Scopus, and Web of Science) to identify studies published between 2000 and 2024 that investigated cCMV infection, diagnostic testing for cCMV, and pediatric hearing loss. Words such as congenital cytomegalovirus, cCMV, screening, and hearing loss were utilized as indicators for article/study inclusion. Abstracts were subsequently reviewed to ensure the accessibility of the article and were excluded if not written in the English language or if the full text was unavailable. The second phase began by reading each article/study that had passed the initial inspection and inclusion criteria. Items that reported the prevalence, characteristics, diagnostic methods, current policies, and/or recommendations for universal cCMV testing in newborns were finally included. Once the final publications were identified, the information and data were compiled, presented, and analyzed by the research team.

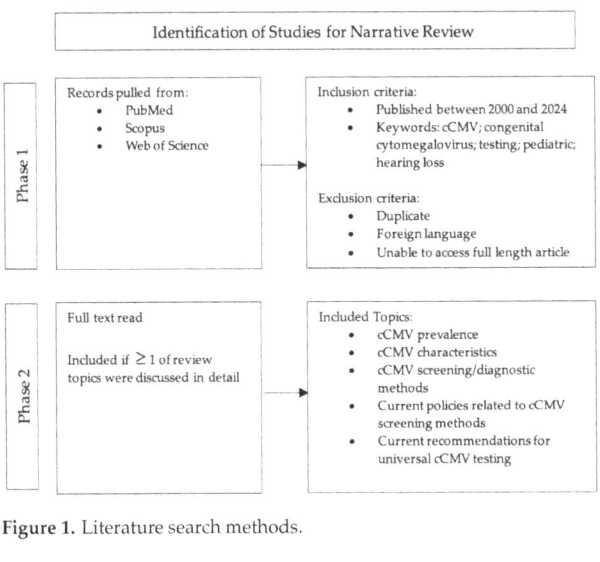

Figure 1. Literature search methods.

This narrative review aimed to highlight the prevalence of cCMV, particularly in the United States; provide insights into the clinical manifestations of cCMV; and summarize the ongoing discussions regarding CMV screening recommendations.

2. Prevalence of cCMV

The impact of cCMV is significant, as it is the leading non-genetic cause of sensorineural hearing loss and a major infectious contributor to neurodevelopmental disabilities in children [5]. Thus, understanding the prevalence of cCMV, particularly the demographics that it affects, is crucial for guiding public health strategies in the prevention and management of at-risk populations.

Globally, cCMV infection has a prevalence at birth varying between 0.2% and 1% (depending on the country's maternal seroprevalence rates) [6]. In the US, this translates to approximately 20,000 to 30,000 infants infected each year [7]. In other developed countries like Canada, those in Western Europe, and Australia, the prevalence of congenital CMV infection is similar, at 0.5% to 0.7% of all live births [8]. Within developing countries, cCMV has an estimated incidence of 0.6–0.7% of all live births [5].

A recent study investigated the impact of advanced maternal age and intrauterine growth restriction on cCMV prevalence. A cohort study from China found that 75 out of 10,993 screened newborns tested positive for cCMV, resulting in an overall prevalence of 0.7%, supporting values found in other studies [9]. Of note, the prevalence of cCMV infections declined with increasing maternal age and increased in preterm infants and those with intrauterine growth limitation, compared to full-term infants and those without these conditions [9].

Some sources cite a disparity in CMV prevalence by maternal race, ethnicity, and geographic location. A recent investigation into previously published cCMV newborn screening studies in the United States found that the adjusted prevalence of cCMV infection, accounting for maternal race and ethnicity, was estimated to be between 4.6 and 4.7 cases per 1000 live births on a national level and to range between 3.9 and 6.5 cases per 1000 across states from 2018 to 2022 [10]. Notably, infants born to non-Hispanic Black mothers had the highest prevalence at 9.3 cases (with a range of 8.2 to 10.5 per 1000), followed by non-Hispanic American Indian and Alaska Native mothers at 8.5 cases (with a range of 2.1 to 33.2 per 1000) [10]. Additionally, the annual prevalence of cCMV infection was consistently highest in the southern states and Alaska [10]. These findings indicate that states with a greater proportion of racial and ethnic minorities have a higher prevalence of cCMV than states with predominantly White populations, and they highlight the importance of cCMV surveillance at the jurisdiction level and the need for tailored and culturally relevant education and prevention strategies for those at higher risk [10].

3. Clinical Presentation

Congenital cytomegalovirus infections typically occur when cytomegalovirus, a member of the Herpesviridae family, is transmitted vertically, through the placenta, from mother to fetus during pregnancy [9,11]. Primary maternal infections occur when a pregnant mother first becomes infected with CMV through close contact with bodily fluids/secretions. This infection subsequently poses a higher risk of vertical transmission than non-primary maternal infections, which are characterized as the reactivation of latent CMV infection or reinfection with a new strain of CMV during pregnancy [7,9,12]. Additionally, cCMV infections resulting from primary maternal infections are more likely to present with symptoms at birth, even when fetal imaging is normal, compared to non-primary maternal infections [9,13].

The presentation of cCMV may be categorized into symptomatic and asymptomatic. Most infected infants present with no clinical features, and the long-term prognosis for those with clinically inapparent infections is excellent [11]. Only about 11% of live infants born with cCMV are symptomatic and present with abnormal clinical findings at birth, with 25% of those infected infants developing sequelae by the age of 2 years [7,14,15]. For those with symptomatic cCMV infections at birth, clinical manifestations can vary and include small for gestational age, intrauterine growth restriction, microcephaly, blueberry muffin rash representing extramedullary hematopoiesis, hepatosplenomegaly, petechiae, thrombocytopenia, jaundice, direct hyperbilirubinemia, elevated alanine aminotransaminase, chorioretinitis, or cerebral calcifications that may be seen as hyperintense signal alterations on MRI [11,13,16,17].

Perhaps the most well-known and feared complication of cCMV is the risk of hearing impairment in the form of SNHL [14,17–19]. Between 20% and 65% of symptomatic infants and 6% and 15% of clinically inapparent at-birth infants will develop SNHL, with severity ranging from mild to profound in unilateral or bilateral ears [7,8,17,20]. This CMV-related hearing loss typically has a fluctuating and progressive course, sometimes resulting in children being undiagnosed until elementary age if not initially apparent at the time of newborn hearing screening [21]. Possible prognostic predictors for hearing outcomes include symptoms of cCMV at birth, failure of neonatal hearing screening, and viral load level in blood [22]. Missed opportunities for the early diagnosis and treatment of cCMV could ultimately lead to severe hearing loss or profound developmental delay [23].

While estimates of long-term sequelae are likely underestimated due to the lack of universal testing at birth and limited follow-up in clinical trials, a retrospective observational study aimed at describing the long-term outcomes of cCMV infection in children identified 61 newborns positive for CMV through a PCR of viral DNA from urine within the first 15 days of life [7,24]. Of the 61 newborns, 20 were diagnosed with sensorineural hearing loss (SNHL), 8 of whom underwent cochlear implantation [24].

4. cCMV Screening Methodology

With early cCMV detection being key in offering treatment and subsequently helping create positive outcomes, many studies have focused on establishing a consistently reliable, feasible, and cost-efficient method to maximize cCMV detection. Methods that have been recently studied and/or implemented in country-wide screening recommendations include perinatal antibody and avidity testing, PCR (polymerase chain reaction) testing of neonatal saliva or urine, and DBS (dried blood spot) testing.

Researchers have studied maternal CMV screening as a predictor of congenital CMV infection in newborns. IgM antibodies that are associated with acute infection can persist for months with IgG antibodies. Therefore, it is difficult to isolate the time of infection. While high IgM with high IgG suggests an infection, it does little to provide a clue as to the infection timeline. This is not a reliable practice for widespread diagnostic utility; however, other testing, such as viral avidity testing, may prove useful.

Viral avidity testing measures the affinity with which IgG antibodies bind to the virus and has been used to assess the risk of fetal transmission in infections such as toxoplasmosis, parvovirus, rubella, and CMV [12]. Reduced viral avidity in recently infected cases (12–18 weeks) acts as an indicator of increased circulating levels of the virus and the risk of fetal transmission, while high avidity indicates an improved immune response, decreased transmission, and higher titers of virus-neutralizing antibodies [12].

A recent study by Raynor et al. investigated the utility of detecting cCMV and predicting SNHL with the concept of avidity [12]. Although a promising concept, the findings showed no significant hearing loss in babies born to CMV-positive mothers, likely because most mothers had a strong immune response (high viral avidity), indicating infection before pregnancy [12]. Consequently, although viral avidity may help to determine whether an infection is recent or from the past, it may not reliably differentiate between congenital infections that pose a risk of SNHL and those that do not, limiting its usefulness in a universal screening protocol.

In neonates, when there is a high suspicion of intrauterine CMV infection, viral isolation and culture from urine or saliva is the traditional standard [14]. The high sensitivity of PCR, alongside the ease of collection and testing of saliva samples, makes this the preferred option [14]. However, the high sensitivity is also associated with a high number of false-positive tests that have been associated with saliva, and any positive saliva result should be subsequently confirmed with a urine sample [14,25]. Importantly, to detect congenital CMV infection, the sample must be collected at birth, as a diagnosis made after the first 2–3 weeks of life could be due to viral transmission through the breast milk of a seropositive mother, possibly contributing to the high rate of false positives [13]. Despite the high false-positive rate, this strategy could provide a convenient and efficient approach to detecting neonatal infection in less developed parts of the world with an otherwise reduced detection capacity [26,27]. However, there have been citations of concern with the cost of the widespread administration of such tests [28]. Targeted urine-filtered screening presents a viable option for neonatal CMV screening when used by itself or as a confirmation exam [29].

Dried blood spot (DBS) testing is a reliable, cost-effective alternative to saliva swabs or urine cultures that may be used to diagnose congenital CMV. This method may offer long-term sample storage and high accuracy (71–100% sensitivity and 99–100% specificity) [30,31]. The broad range of sensitivity offers some controversy on whether this method could dependably offer an accurate diagnosis if implemented universally [32]. However, those who support this method point to the ability of DBS PCR testing to be integrated into existing newborn screening protocols, encouraging the utility of this option for neonatal screening and diagnosis [25]. Previous studies have shown the utility of Guthrie card DBS samples, positively identifying all neonates with a cCMV infection, including those who were asymptomatic and without some degree of hearing impairment [23]. DBS screening for cCMV could be adequate in clinical practice and presents a practical, viable approach for universal mass screening [33].

Some studies have investigated the benefit of a combined, comprehensive program that integrates physiologic, genetic, and cCMV screening alongside universal newborn hearing screening [34]. By identifying at-risk infants who would otherwise go unnoticed through conventional methods, this strategy ensures early intervention, which is paramount for speech and cognitive growth and development. Additionally, obtaining etiological data early on enables personalized treatment planning, removing ambiguity from families and clinicians. By maximizing diagnostics, this strategy may also limit the loss to follow-up of children, ensuring that they have adequate care. Furthermore, the early identification of risk factors may reduce the need for costly repeated testing throughout later childhood, ultimately optimizing healthcare resources, with improved long-term outcomes among affected children. In summary, this strategy could work to enhance the early detection of hearing loss, provide etiologic insights, improve follow-up rates, and reduce long-term testing costs [34].

5. Targeted Neonatal Screening

According to international standards, targeted screening is currently indicated either when a newborn fails their hearing screening protocol, for example, the Transient Evoked Otoacoustic Emissions (TEOAE) assessment, or when a newborn presents with findings suggestive of cCMV infection, such as thrombocytopenia, jaundice, or microcephaly [12,15,35]. If either indication is met, a newborn will undergo more "targeted" testing, typically through the detection of viral DNA by PCR of a saliva or urine sample [35–37]. A neonate with confirmed cCMV and hearing loss can then be offered antiviral therapy for implementation within their first month of life [38].

Currently recommended by the American Academy of Audiology, as well as the Newborn Hearing Screening Working Group of the National Coordinating Center for the Regional Genetics Networks, targeted cCMV screening is the most implemented screening measure to detect cCMV infections in newborns [11,16,35]. Its use is seen widely in the United States, Canada, the United Kingdom, Europe, and Australia [35,39,40].

Designed as a prospective survey of birth hospitals performing early cCMV testing, the NIH ValEAR clinical trial was a study aimed at determining the positivity rate of the three main approaches: universal CMV testing, hearing-targeted CMV testing (HT-cCMV), and delayed targeted dried blood spot (DBS) testing [8]. The researchers found that the positivity rates of cCMV among the three different approaches were 0.5%, 1.5%, and 7.3%, respectively, with results consistent with cohort studies reported in the literature [8]. The largest group of infants (n = 9017) underwent HT-cCMV screening, and this group comprised the greatest number of detected CMV infections at n = 132 [8].

A recent study investigated parents' perceptions of such testing and found that families felt as though it was feasible, acceptable, and generally a good idea to test the neonate for congenital infection [41]. Further investigation into the associated cost indicated that implementing targeted cCMV screening is both feasible and financially viable, with minimal cost differences compared to non-screening [42].

Targeted screening is widely endorsed as the standard practice, whereas universal screening, though less common, is increasingly viewed as the best approach for identifying children with cCMV [35,43].

6. Current State and Perceptions of Universal Neonatal Screening

Universal neonatal screening may ultimately lead to the early diagnosis of cCMV, thus catching the infection early and offering an opportunity to treat and potentially avoid a devastating and debilitating diagnosis of SNHL. This may ultimately improve both linguistic skills and cognitive development in the affected population [44]. Coupled with the proven effectiveness and increase in accessibility, the proven benefits of early identification and intervention on auditory outcomes are undoubtable [44,45]. Current international guidelines maintain recommendations for cCMV screening for infants who fail universal newborn hearing screening [38]. However, this presents a missed opportunity to accurately diagnose those who will ultimately present with late-onset hearing loss, secondary to the CMV [46–48]. Perhaps one of the most significant barriers to implementing universal neonatal cCMV screening is the cost. A recent study by Saito et al. comparing the direct and long-term care costs of universal and targeted screening suggested that, despite higher incremental costs, universal screening is ultimately more cost-effective than targeted screening [49].

Despite cCMV infection meeting many of the criteria for a universal screening program according to the WHO (World Health Organization), and a multitude of studies trialing such a program in hospital centers with promising results, no country has yet implemented such a program [6].

6.1. Within the USA

The proven benefits of early identification and intervention (at <6 months of age) in terms of language outcomes and communication have confirmed the effectiveness and utility of universal cCMV neonatal screening. Further, recent studies support the greater overall cost savings and maximal opportunity to deliver targeted medical intervention to those in need [46,50,51]. The cCMV screening landscape varies across the United States (Figure 2). Although CMV is more prevalent than many conditions included in newborn screening programs, only a few states in the country (Texas, Minnesota, and New York) have adopted universal cCMV screening policies to date [7]. In other states, screening follows international recommendations and is often targeted based on hospital or state policies, with testing primarily conducted in infants presenting specific clinical indicators, such as failed hearing screening, microcephaly, a low birth weight, and thrombocytopenia [7]. Despite the variation in current screening protocols, a recent study performed in the US confirmed that the implementation of state newborn hearing screening programs corresponded to increasing diagnosis rates of cCMV with hearing loss (0.87 [0.51–1.22],

$p < 0.001$) [52]. Additionally, there were significant increases in early CMV detection in both symptomatic (0.68 [0.37–0.99], $p < 0.001$) and asymptomatic (0.18 [0.03–0.32], $p = 0.02$) neonates [52]. Notably, this increase in diagnosis rates could also be attributed to an increase in education and awareness about this impactful congenital infection.

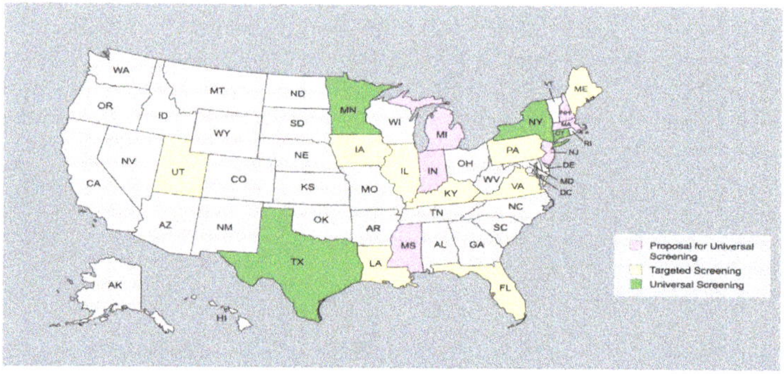

Figure 2. cCMV screening landscape across the United States.

While newborn hearing screening has significantly improved early CMV detection, those positive for infection but failing to present with the "typical" clinical symptoms may be undetected, delaying crucial intervention.

6.2. Around the World

Richard et al. conducted a study in France to characterize the implementation of universal screening for cCMV in neonates via a CMV PCR saliva test, ultimately testing 98.1% of infants in the study period, and they found an infection prevalence of 0.4%; this investigation also found that screening had a high parental acceptance rate and that testing administration was feasible [6]. Further, only 38% of newborns presented with signs characteristic of infection, supporting the notion that, in the absence of universal screening, most cases would remain undiagnosed [6].

As previously discussed, another option for congenital CMV detection is utilizing materials that would otherwise be discarded with DBS screening. In a recent study of 433 infants that assessed the utility of discarded umbilical cord blood, 2 (0.5%) tested positive for CMV in their cord blood, with 1 showing symptoms; both infants had mothers who previously had CMV but showed no recent infection [53].

The Tuscany region of Italy has seen some success with the implementation of universal cCMV screening protocols. Coupling TEOAE and AABR screening with auditory follow-up may positively improve rehabilitation results in terms of hearing abilities and linguistic and communicative skills [54].

In England, targeted surveillance has traditionally been utilized as the primary method for monitoring children who may be at risk of developing hearing loss, regardless of the hearing screening outcome [55]. Currently, the JCIH (Joint Committee on Infant Hearing) maintains the recommendation of monitoring risk factors to detect postnatal hearing loss by 3 months in cases of CMV [56]. Although it is important to diagnose cCMV-associated hearing loss and monitor these children, multiple follow-up visits for monitoring can place excessive strain on families and audiology services [55]. This could leave an opportunity for universal screening to help bridge the gap.

In Japan, a recent investigation utilized PCR screening of urine from 23, 368 newborns to screen for cCMV infection. In addition to the PCR analysis, newborn hearing screening (automated auditory brainstem response (AABR) testing) was conducted within 5 days of birth to examine the incidence of cCMV infection and SNHL, respectively [56]. The study determined that the incidence of late-onset SNHL and neurodevelopmental disorders is associated with and may be predicted by an increase in urinary CMV viral load [57]. This investigation helps support the idea that quantitative viral load measurements may help to more accurately detect the incidence of cCMV infection.

A recent study performed in Australia examined parental opinions on a targeted saliva swab for cCMV from 2019 to 2020 as authorities considered the option of placing screening protocols in the hands of parents [38]. Although the results found that the swab offered a non-invasive screening technique that was generally well received by parents and easily delivered, a high false-positive rate could increase anxiety and uneasiness [38]. This could potentially be mitigated by increasing public knowledge of cCMV and completing the swab at the hospital to reduce the risk of false positives from completing the swab incorrectly or breastmilk contamination [38]. Other studies support the potential for saliva PCR testing to be used in screening protocols as a feasible and effective method, whether that is with the assistance of parental or healthcare worker administration [57].

Countries like Norway have created registries to collect data and set quality standards for newborn hearing screening and early intervention [58]. These registries track key metrics, including the rate of false positives in hearing tests, CMV testing within three weeks for infants who fail screening, the confirmation of hearing status by three months, and the start of intervention within three months of diagnosis [59]. Having registries such as these could help identify the most suitable screening methodology that could be adopted and implemented worldwide.

In Spain, the Commission for the Early Detection of Hearing Loss (CODEPEH) has encouraged universal neonatal hearing screening [59]. This approach helps prevent false negatives in individuals who do not have risk factors for congenital hearing loss, which accounts for 60% of cases [59]. This screening may utilize objective methods such as otoacoustic emissions or automatic auditory evoked potentials (AEPs) and allow for the subsequent testing of cCMV by a PCR of urine and saliva, as well as the opportunity to deliver life-altering treatment [59].

A study based in Germany screened 6102 newborns for cCMV using buccal swabs within the first three days of life, with confirmatory testing for those who tested positive, while ensuring measures to prevent false positives from breast milk [60]. This research highlights a highly effective cCMV screening strategy using eNAT™ medium and quantitative PCR, supporting centralized pooled saliva testing while emphasizing the need for clinical follow-up to establish a viral load threshold for negligible late-onset CMV disease risk [60].

Some studies have investigated the efficacy of establishing universal cCMV testing in premature infants born before 33 weeks of gestation. Out of 549 urine samples/infants identified, none were positive for CMV DNA, suggesting that a combination of failed hearing tests with universal screening could more closely select for and identify those positive for cCMV that may benefit from appropriate treatment [61,62].

In resource-limited geographic locations, there have been some questions regarding the feasibility of implementing universal screening in an already resource-strained landscape. However, studies in Northern India offer positive reassurance that this is possible, with study findings demonstrating the feasibility and value of simultaneous newborn screening for both cCMV and hearing loss in a resource-limited setting [63].

7. Discussion

Regardless of screening protocols, the implementation of regular, strategic follow-up plans remains crucial for ensuring timely intervention and optimal outcomes for affected infants [64,65]. Consistent monitoring can help identify late-onset complications and enable early therapeutic measures, ultimately improving long-term prognoses.

Two expert groups, the International Congenital Cytomegalovirus Recommendations Group (ICCRG) and the European Society for Pediatric Infectious Diseases (ESPID), strongly advocate for antiviral therapy in newborns with moderate-to-severe symptomatic congenital CMV (cCMV), based on robust evidence from randomized controlled trials (RCTs) [66]. This treatment approach has been shown to mitigate short-term and potentially long-term hearing deterioration, reinforcing its role in clinical management. However, a significant challenge lies in the fact that the majority of cCMV cases present mild or subclinical manifestations, including isolated sensorineural hearing loss (SNHL), which often remain undetected in the absence of targeted screening [59,67]. As a result, treatment recommendations vary across guidelines [58], reflecting the ongoing debate regarding the necessity and efficacy of antiviral therapy in these cases.

Despite these uncertainties, the benefits of early detection and intervention, such as hearing amplification, speech therapy, and other supportive measures, are increasingly evident for children at risk of late-onset SNHL. Universal screening programs play a pivotal role in identifying these at-risk infants, allowing for timely intervention that may significantly enhance developmental and auditory outcomes. A universal hearing screening protocol that can be easily integrated into routine newborn screening labs would be ideal and perhaps offer the most consistent rates of early cCMV detection, as shown in recent pilot programs [68]. Integrating CMV diagnostics into routine newborn screening workflows may not only substantially increase detection rates but also ensure timely care pathways in an interdisciplinary manner and a multifactorial approach.

Looking forward, the future of cCMV diagnostics is braced for scientific, medical, and technological advancement. First, the development of rapid, high-sensitivity molecular assays that can be seamlessly integrated into existing newborn screening platforms will revolutionize the means of cCMV detection. Rapid PCR analyses of saliva and dried blood spots have previously been studied in terms of their utility for early detection, offering success while also identifying areas for improvement. It will remain important that the method(s) utilized for early cCMV detection are implemented as low-cost, efficient options with high reproducibility and specificity. Additionally, as artificial learning algorithms continue to become intertwined within the field of healthcare, they may be used to assist the diagnosing and managing clinician. With the potential to identify subtle clinical patterns, enhance risk stratification, support individualized follow-up plans, and connect families with specific resources, this may act as a key resource in maximizing early cCMV detection and optimizing outcomes. Further, continued investigation into the human genome could be important for genomic and proteomic profiling that could offer key clues to novel biomarkers that may be used for the early detection and ultimate prognosis of complications related to cCMV.

The continued sharing of trials related to diagnostic methods will continue to be useful in shaping consistent screening and treatment practices across healthcare systems worldwide. These advancements, combined with continued advocacy and public health investment, have the potential to transform cCMV from a frequently missed diagnosis into a condition that is systematically identified, monitored, and managed from the earliest days of life.

In sum, a comprehensive approach that combines universal screening with structured follow-up and evolving diagnostic technologies is essential for optimizing the care and outcomes of infants with cCMV. Future advances in diagnostics and individualized therapeutic models offer a promising outlook, working to close the current gaps in detection and treatment and improving the quality of life of affected children and their families.

8. Conclusions

Because there is no effective CMV vaccine available to date, congenital cytomegalovirus remains a significant global health burden, particularly affecting children of mothers from lower socioeconomic backgrounds. Although most cases of cCMV are asymptomatic, nearly 25% of infants will go on to develop adverse neurodevelopmental outcomes, including sensorineural hearing loss; vision impairment; and speech, language, and learning delays. Apart from educating women on how to reduce their risk of contracting CMV during pregnancy, CMV screening programs are currently the best preventative care measure in improving the outcomes of children with CMV, as they allow for early detection and, more importantly, timely intervention with antiviral therapy. Targeted screening is currently the standard of care due to its practicality and feasibility. However, in the future, and if infrastructure improves, we may expect more states and countries to adopt universal CMV screening programs to identify all those with CMV infections, including infants who would develop hearing loss later in life.

9. Future Directions

Future policy and research initiatives must aim to improve universal CMV screening programs to detect and intervene early for all such affected infants, including those at risk of late-onset disease. Although targeted screening is the present norm because of its practicality, advancements in technology and healthcare infrastructure may, in the future, make universal screening a more functional option. Large-scale comparisons of the cost-effectiveness and long-term efficacy of universal screening will be most important to guide policy changes and broader implementation. Refining the diagnostic tools to make them more accurate and efficient at screening, such as point-of-care testing or newborn screening panel tests, also has the potential to integrate early detection into streamlined procedures.

In parallel, continued investment in vaccine research remains a critical priority in the fight against congenital CMV. The development of an effective CMV vaccine could significantly reduce the incidence of congenital infections and alleviate the long-term neurodevelopmental burden associated with the virus. Ongoing clinical trials exploring potential vaccine candidates must be supported through sustained funding and global collaboration to accelerate progress. Furthermore, expanding public health initiatives to educate women of childbearing age and families on CMV transmission prevention strategies remains essential. Combining enhanced screening programs, vaccine development, and widespread education efforts can create a comprehensive approach to mitigating the impact of congenital CMV on a global scale.

Author Contributions: A.C.: conceptualization, methodology, literature review, formal analysis, investigation, writing—original draft preparation, writing—review and editing; A.J.: literature review, formal analysis, investigation, writing—original draft preparation, writing—review and editing; E.W.: Conceptualization, methodology, literature review; T.L.F.: writing—review and editing; G.M.: Conceptualization, methodology, visualization, supervision of all project processes and drafts, writing—original draft preparation, writing—review and editing. All authors have read and agreed to the published version of the manuscript.

Funding: This research received no external funding.

Institutional Review Board Statement: Not applicable.

Informed Consent Statement: Not applicable.

Data Availability Statement: No new data were created or analyzed in this study. Data sharing does not apply to this article.

Acknowledgments: The authors would like to thank the LSUHS Otolaryngology and Head and Neck Surgery departments for their support in publishing this review.

Conflicts of Interest: The authors declare no conflicts of interest.

References

1. Pasternak, Y.; Ziv, L.; Attias, J.; Amir, J.; Bilavsky, E. Valganciclovir Is Beneficial in Children with Congenital Cytomegalovirus and Isolated Hearing Loss. *J. Pediatr.* **2018**, *199*, 166–170. [CrossRef] [PubMed]
2. Chung, P.K.; Schornagel, F.A.J.; Soede, W.; Van Zwet, E.W.; Kroes, A.C.M.; Oudesluys-Murphy, A.M.; Vossen, A.C.T. Valganciclovir in Infants with Hearing Loss and Clinically Inapparent Congenital Cytomegalovirus Infection: A Nonrandomized Controlled Trial. *J. Pediatr.* **2024**, *268*, 113945. [CrossRef] [PubMed]
3. Leruez-Ville, M.; Chatzakis, C.; Lilleri, D.; Blazquez-Gamero, D.; Alarcon, A.; Bourgon, N.; Foulon, I.; Fourgeaud, J.; Gonce, A.; Jones, C.E.; et al. Consensus recommendation for prenatal, neonatal and postnatal management of congenital cytomegalovirus infection from the European congenital infection initiative (ECCI). *Lancet Reg. Health Eur.* **2024**, *40*, 100892. [CrossRef] [PubMed] [PubMed Central]
4. De Cuyper, E.; Acke, F.; Keymeulen, A.; Dhooge, I. The Effect of (Val)ganciclovir on Hearing in Congenital Cytomegalovirus: A Systematic Review. *Laryngoscope* **2022**, *132*, 2241–2250. [CrossRef]
5. Marsico, C.; Kimberlin, D. Congenital Cytomegalovirus infection: Advances and challenges in diagnosis, prevention and treatment. *Ital. J. Pediatr.* **2017**, *43*, 38. [CrossRef]
6. Letamendia-Richard, E.; Périllaud-Dubois, C.; de La Guillonnière, L.; Thouard, I.; Cordier, A.G.; Roque-Afonso, A.M.; de Luca, D.; Benachi, A.; Vauloup-Fellous, C. Universal newborn screening for congenital cytomegalovirus infection: Feasibility and relevance in a French type-III maternity cohort. *BJOG Int. J. Obstet. Gynaecol.* **2022**, *129*, 291–299. [CrossRef]
7. Stark, A.; Crooks, C.M.; Permar, S.R.; Weimer, K.E.D. Neonatal Cytomegalovirus Infection: Advocacy, Legislation, and Changing Practice. *Clin. Perinatol.* **2025**, *52*, 115–132. [CrossRef]
8. Orb, Q.T.; Pesch, M.; Allen, C.M.; Wilkes, A.; Ahmad, I.; Alfonso, K.; Antonio, S.M.; Mithal, L.B.; Brinkmeirer, J.V.; Carvalho, D.; et al. Congenital Cytomegalovirus Testing Outcomes From the ValEAR Trial. *Otolaryngol.-Head Neck Surg.* **2024**, *170*, 1430–1441. [CrossRef]
9. Wang, S.; Wang, T.; Zhang, W.; Liu, X.; Wang, X.; Wang, H.; He, X.; Zhang, S.; Xu, S.; Jia, X.; et al. Cohort study on maternal cytomegalovirus seroprevalence and prevalence and clinical manifestations of congenital infection in China. *Medicine* **2017**, *96*, e6007. [CrossRef]
10. Lutz, C.S.; Schleiss, M.R.; Fowler, K.B.; Lanzieri, T.M. Updated National and State-Specific Prevalence of Congenital Cytomegalovirus Infection, United States, 2018–2022. *J. Public Health Manag. Pract.* **2025**, *31*, 234–243. [CrossRef]
11. Nishikawa, J.K.; Sánchez, P.J. Congenital Cytomegalovirus Infection and Hearing Loss: It's Time to Screen. *Otol. Neurotol.* **2024**, *45*, e702–e709. [CrossRef] [PubMed]
12. Raynor, E.M.; Martin, H.L.; Poehlein, E.; Lee, H.J.; Lantos, P. Impact of maternal cytomegalovirus seroconversion on newborn and childhood hearing loss. *Laryngoscope Investig. Otolaryngol.* **2022**, *7*, 1626–1633. [CrossRef] [PubMed]
13. Zhang, L.; Li, Z.; Han, X.; Du, H.; Cao, Y.; Liu, Y.; Wang, W. Association between Congenital Cytomegalovirus Infection and Brain Injury in Neonates: A Meta-analysis of Cohort Studies. *Behav. Neurol.* **2021**, *2021*, 9603660. [CrossRef] [PubMed]
14. Lazzarotto, T.; Blázquez-Gamero, D.; Delforge, M.; Foulon, I.; Luck, S.; Modrow, S.; Leruez-Ville, M. Congenital Cytomegalovirus Infection: A Narrative Review of the Issues in Screening and Management From a Panel of European Experts. *Front. Pediatr.* **2020**, *8*, 13. [CrossRef]
15. Gaur, P.; Ffrench-Constant, S.; Kachramanoglou, C.; Lyall, H.; Jan, W. Is it not time for international guidelines to combat congenital cytomegalovirus infection? A review of central nervous system manifestations. *Clin. Radiol.* **2020**, *75*, 644.e7–644.e16. [CrossRef]
16. Suarez, D.; Nielson, C.; McVicar, S.B.; Sidesinger, M.; Ostrander, B.; O'Brien, E.; Ampofo, K.; Ling, C.Y.; Miner, L.J.; Park, A.H. Analysis of an Expanded Targeted Early Cytomegalovirus Testing Program. *Otolaryngol.-Head Neck Surg.* **2023**, *169*, 679–686. [CrossRef]
17. Cushing, S.L.; Purcell, P.L.; Papaiaonnou, V.; Neghandi, J.; Daien, M.; Blaser, S.I.; Ertl-Wagner, B.; Wagner, M.; Sheng, M.; James, A.L.; et al. Hearing Instability in Children with Congenital Cytomegalovirus: Evidence and Neural Consequences. *Laryngoscope* **2022**, *132*, S1–S24. [CrossRef]
18. Pollick, S.A.; Mansour, Y.; Pesch, M.H. Newborn congenital cytomegalovirus screening and hearing outcomes: A systematic review of current literature. *Curr. Opin. Otolaryngol. Head Neck Surg.* **2024**, *32*, 329–338. [CrossRef]
19. Dedhia, K.; Graham, E.; Park, A. Hearing Loss and Failed Newborn Hearing Screen. *Clin. Perinatol.* **2018**, *45*, 629–643. [CrossRef]

20. Tapasak, B.; Cronkite, D.A.; Hustedt-Mai, A.R.; Morlet, T.M.; Parkes, W.J.; Maul, T.M.; Parkes, W.J.; Maul, T.M.; Pritchett, C.V. Hearing outcomes in children with Congenital Cytomegalovirus: A multi-center, single-enterprise experience. *Int. J Pediatr. Otorhinolaryngol.* **2022**, *163*, 111376. [CrossRef]
21. Friis, I.J.; Aaberg, K.; Edholm, B. Causes of hearing loss and implantation age in a cohort of Danish pediatric cochlear implant recipients. *Int. J. Pediatr. Otorhinolaryngol.* **2023**, *171*, 111640. [CrossRef] [PubMed]
22. Lo, T.H.; Lin, P.H.; Hsu, W.C.; Tsao, P.N.; Liu, T.C.; Yang, T.H.; Hsu, C.J.; Huang, L.M.; Lu, C.Y.; Wu, C.C. Prognostic determinants of hearing outcomes in children with congenital cytomegalovirus infection. *Sci. Rep.* **2022**, *12*, 5219. [CrossRef] [PubMed]
23. Shahar-Nissan, K.; Oikawa Tepperberg, M.; Mendelson, E.; Bilavsky, E. Retrospective identification of congenital cytomegalovirus infection using dried blood samples-missed opportunities and lessons. *J. Clin. Virol.* **2022**, *152*, 105186. [CrossRef]
24. Forli, F.; Capobianco, S.; Berrettini, S.; Bruschini, L.; Lorenzoni, F.; Fiori, S.; Lazzerini, F. Long-term outcomes of congenital cytomegalovirus infection in children early identified by extended hearing-targeted screening. *Int. J. Pediatr. Otorhinolaryngol.* **2024**, *184*, 112070. [CrossRef]
25. Schleiss, M.R.; Blázquez-Gamero, D. Universal newborn screening for congenital cytomegalovirus infection. *Lancet Child Adolesc. Health* **2025**, *9*, 57–70. [CrossRef]
26. Ari-Even Roth, D.; Lubin, D.; Kuint, J.; Teperberg-Oikawa, M.; Mendelson, E.; Strauss, T.; Barkai, G. Contribution of targeted saliva screening for congenital CMV-related hearing loss in newborns who fail hearing screening. *Arch. Dis. Child. Fetal Neonatal Ed.* **2017**, *102*, F519–F524. [CrossRef]
27. Izquierdo, G.; Farfan, M.J.; Villavicencio, L.; Montecinos, L.; Tarque, F.; Acevedo, W.; Reyes, R.; Guerra, C.; Araya, L.; Sepulveda, B.; et al. Optimizing congenital cytomegalovirus detection by pool testing in saliva by a rapid molecular test. *Eur. J. Pediatr.* **2023**, *182*, 5131–5136. [CrossRef]
28. Jin, Y.; Liu, X.; Chen, S.; Xiang, J.; Peng, Z.; Sun, Y. Analysis of the Results of Cytomegalovirus Testing Combined with Genetic Testing in Children with Congenital Hearing Loss. *J. Clin. Med.* **2022**, *11*, 5335. [CrossRef]
29. Koyano, S.; Morioka, I.; Oka, A.; Moriuchi, H.; Asano, K.; Ito, Y.; Yoshikawa, T.; Yamada, H.; Suzutani, T.; Inoue, N.; et al. Congenital cytomegalovirus in Japan: More than 2 year follow up of infected newborns. *Pediatr. Int.* **2018**, *60*, 57–62. [CrossRef]
30. Barbi, M.; Binda, S.; Caroppo, S. Diagnosis of congenital CMV infection via dried blood spots. *Rev. Med. Virol.* **2006**, *16*, 385–392. [CrossRef]
31. Yoshimura, H.; Okubo, T.; Shinagawa, J.; Nishio, S.Y.; Takumi, Y.; Usami, S.I. Epidemiology, aetiology and diagnosis of congenital hearing loss via hearing screening of 153913 newborns. *Int. J. Epidemiol.* **2024**, *53*, dyae052. [CrossRef] [PubMed]
32. Dobbie, A.M. Evaluation and management of cytomegalovirus-associated congenital hearing loss. *Curr. Opin. Otolaryngol. Head Neck Surg.* **2017**, *25*, 390–395. [CrossRef] [PubMed]
33. Moteki, H.; Isaka, Y.; Inaba, Y.; Motobayashi, M.; Nishio, S.Y.; Ohira, S.; Yano, T.; Iwasaki, S.; Shiozawa, T.; Koike, K.; et al. A rational approach to identifying newborns with hearing loss caused by congenital cytomegalovirus infection by dried blood spot screening. *Acta Oto-Laryngol.* **2018**, *138*, 708–712. [CrossRef] [PubMed]
34. Shearer, A.E.; Shen, J.; Amr, S.; Morton, C.C.; Smith, R.J. A proposal for comprehensive newborn hearing screening to improve identification of deaf and hard-of-hearing children. *Genet. Med.* **2019**, *21*, 2614–2630. [CrossRef]
35. Gantt, S. Newborn cytomegalovirus screening: Is this the new standard? *Curr. Opin. Otolaryngol. Head Neck Surg.* **2023**, *31*, 382–387. [CrossRef]
36. Fourgeaud, J.; Boithias, C.; Walter-Nicolet, E.; Kermorvant, E.; Couderc, S.; Parat, S.; Pol, C.; Mousset, C.; Bussieres, L.; Guilleminot, T.; et al. Performance of Targeted Congenital Cytomegalovirus Screening in Newborns Failing Universal Hearing Screening: A Multicenter Study. *Pediatr. Infect. Dis. J.* **2022**, *41*, 478–481. [CrossRef]
37. Blázquez-Gamero, D.; Soriano-Ramos, M.; Vicente, M.; Pallás-Alonso, C.R.; Pérez-Rivilla, A.; García-Álvarez, M.; Martin, M.T.P.; Freire, X.; Vergas, J.D.; Martinez De Aragon, A.; et al. Prevalence and Clinical Manifestations of Congenital Cytomegalovirus Infection in a Screening Program in Madrid (PICCSA Study). *Pediatr. Infect. Dis. J.* **2020**, *39*, 1050–1056. [CrossRef]
38. Webb, E.; Hodgson, J.; Gillespie, A.N.; Jones, C.A.; Poulakis, Z.; Wong, J.; Sung, V. Hearing Screening for Congenital CytoMegaloVirus-Exploring Parents' Experiences of Completing Targeted Congenital Cytomegalovirus Screening at the Time of Their Infants' Newborn Hearing Screening. *J. Clin. Med.* **2024**, *13*, 4367. [CrossRef]
39. Haller, T.; Shoup, A.; Park, A.H. Should hearing targeted screening for congenital cytomegalovirus infection Be implemented? *Int. J. Pediatr. Otorhinolaryngol.* **2020**, *134*, 110055. [CrossRef]
40. Bartlett, A.W.; Hall, B.M.; Palasanthiran, P.; McMullan, B.; Shand, A.W.; Rawlinson, W.D. Recognition, treatment, and sequelae of congenital cytomegalovirus in Australia: An observational study. *J. Clin. Virol.* **2018**, *108*, 121–125. [CrossRef]
41. Webb, E.; Gillespie, A.N.; Poulakis, Z.; Gartland, T.; Buttery, J.; Casalaz, D.; Daley, A.J.; Donath, S.; Gwee, A.; Jacobs, S.E.; et al. Feasibility and acceptability of targeted salivary cytomegalovirus screening through universal newborn hearing screening. *J. Paediatr. Child Health* **2022**, *58*, 288–294. [CrossRef] [PubMed]

42. Beswick, R.; David, M.; Higashi, H.; Thomas, D.; Nourse, C.; Koh, G.; Koorts, P.; Jardine, L.A.; Clark, J.E. Integration of congenital cytomegalovirus screening within a newborn hearing screening programme. *J. Paediatr. Child Health.* **2019**, *55*, 1381–1388. [CrossRef] [PubMed]
43. Ronner, E.A.; Glovsky, C.K.; Herrmann, B.S.; Woythaler, M.A.; Pasternack, M.S.; Cohen, M.S. Congenital Cytomegalovirus Targeted Screening Implementation and Outcomes: A Retrospective Chart Review. *Otolaryngol.-Head Neck Surg.* **2022**, *167*, 178–182. [CrossRef] [PubMed]
44. Paludetti, G.; Conti, G.; Di Nardo, W.; De Corso, E.; Rolesi, R.; Picciotti, P.; Fetoni, A.R. Infant hearing loss: From diagnosis to therapy Official Report of XXI Conference of Italian Society of Pediatric Otorhinolaryngology. *Acta Otorhinolaryngol. Ital.* **2012**, *32*, 347–370.
45. Goderis, J.; Keymeulen, A.; Smets, K.; Van Hoecke, H.; De Leenheer, E.; Boudewyns, A.; Desloovere, C.; Kuhweide, R.; Muylle, M.; Royackers, L.; et al. Hearing in Children with Congenital Cytomegalovirus Infection: Results of a Longitudinal Study. *J. Pediatr.* **2016**, *172*, 110–115.e2. [CrossRef]
46. Minami, S.B.; Yamanobe, Y.; Nakano, A.; Sakamoto, H.; Masuda, S.; Takiguchi, T.; Katsunuma, S.; Sugiuchi, T.; Morita, N.; Kaga, K.; et al. A High Risk of Missing Congenital Cytomegalovirus-Associated Hearing Loss through Newborn Hearing Screening in Japan. *J. Clin. Med.* **2021**, *10*, 5056. [CrossRef]
47. Jenks, C.M.; Mithal, L.B.; Hoff, S.R. Early Identification and Management of Congenital Cytomegalovirus. *Otolaryngol. Clin. N. Am.* **2021**, *54*, 1117–1127. [CrossRef]
48. Lu, C.Y.; Tsao, P.N.; Ke, Y.Y.; Lin, Y.H.; Lin, Y.H.; Hung, C.C.; Su, Y.N.; Hsu, W.C.; Hseih, W.S.; Huang, L.M.; et al. Concurrent Hearing, Genetic, and Cytomegalovirus Screening in Newborns, Taiwan. *J. Pediatr.* **2018**, *199*, 144–150.e1. [CrossRef]
49. Saito, H.; Sakai, K.; Tanaka, M.; Konomura, K.; Suzuki, M.; Tajima, G.; Hoshino, E. Economic evaluation of newborn screening for congenital cytomegalovirus infection: A systematic review. *Eur. J. Pediatr.* **2025**, *184*, 123. [CrossRef]
50. Williams, E.J.; Gray, J.; Luck, S.; Atkinson, C.; Embleton, N.D.; Kadambari, S.; Davis, A.; Griffiths, P.; Sharland, M.; Berrington, J.E.; et al. First estimates of the potential cost and cost saving of protecting childhood hearing from damage caused by congenital CMV infection. *Arch. Dis. Child. Fetal Neonatal Ed.* **2015**, *100*, F501–F506. [CrossRef]
51. Gantt, S.; Dionne, F.; Kozak, F.K.; Goshen, O.; Goldfarb, D.M.; Park, A.H.; Boppana, S.B.; Fowler, K. Cost-effectiveness of Universal and Targeted Newborn Screening for Congenital Cytomegalovirus Infection. *JAMA Pediatr.* **2016**, *170*, 1173–1180. [CrossRef] [PubMed]
52. So, R.J.; Noij, K.S.; Wang, J.; Walsh, J.; Gourin, C.G.; Jenks, C.M. National and Regional Trends in Congenital Cytomegalovirus Infection From 1998 to 2019. *Otolaryngol.-Head Neck Surg.* **2025**, *172*, 1409–1417. [CrossRef] [PubMed]
53. Theiler, R.; Caliendo, A.; Pargman, S.; Raynor, B.; Berga, S.; McPheeters, M.; Jamieson, D.J. Umbilical cord blood screening for cytomegalovirus DNA by quantitative PCR. *J. Clin. Virol.* **2006**, *37*, 313–316. [CrossRef] [PubMed]
54. Berrettini, S.; Ghirri, P.; Lazzerini, F.; Lenzi, G.; Forli, F. Newborn hearing screening protocol in tuscany region. *Ital. J. Pediatr.* **2017**, *43*, 82. [CrossRef]
55. Geal Dor, M.; Gross, M.; Adelman, C. Follow-Up of Neonatal Hearing Screening in the Risk Factor Group for Hearing Loss: Results from a Tertiary Medical Center. *Children* **2024**, *11*, 1336. [CrossRef]
56. Yamaguchi, A.; Oh-Ishi, T.; Arai, T.; Sakata, H.; Adachi, N.; Asanuma, S.; Oguma, E.; Kimoto, H.; Matsumoto, J.; Fujita, H.; et al. Screening for seemingly healthy newborns with congenital cytomegalovirus infection by quantitative real-time polymerase chain reaction using newborn urine: An observational study. *BMJ Open* **2017**, *7*, e013810. [CrossRef]
57. Barkai, G.; Ari-Even Roth, D.; Barzilai, A.; Tepperberg-Oikawa, M.; Mendelson, E.; Hildesheimer, M.; Kuint, J. Universal neonatal cytomegalovirus screening using saliva—Report of clinical experience. *J. Clin. Virol.* **2014**, *60*, 361–366. [CrossRef]
58. Mattsson, T.S.; Nilsen, A.H.; Wennberg, S. Establishment of the Norwegian hearing register for children. *Front. Hum. Neurosci.* **2024**, *18*, 1400005. [CrossRef]
59. Gutiérrez Posso, J.D.; Anta Escuredo, J.A.; Aguirre Unceta-Barrenechea, A.; Zabala López de Maturana, J.A. Importance of congenital cytomegalovirus in the neonatal hearing screening program. *Acta Otorrinolaringol. Esp. (Engl. Ed.).* **2023**, *74*, 346–351. [CrossRef]
60. Nagel, A.; Dimitrakopoulou, E.; Teig, N.; Kern, P.; Lücke, T.; Michna, D.; Korn, K.; Steininger, P.; Shahada, K.; Neumann, K.; et al. Characterization of a universal screening approach for congenital CMV infection based on a highly-sensitive, quantitative, multiplex real-time PCR assay. *PLoS ONE* **2020**, *15*, e0227143. [CrossRef]
61. Melamed, R.; Shemer-Avni, Y.; Shany, E.; Kurtzman, L.; Gorali, R.; Landau, D. Targeted and universal screen in term and preterm infants for congenital CMV infection. *Infect. Dis.* **2020**, *52*, 730–735. [CrossRef] [PubMed]
62. Lorenzoni, F.; Lunardi, S.; Liumbruno, A.; Ferri, G.; Madrigali, V.; Fiorentini, E.; Forli, F.; Berrettini, S.; Boldrini, A.; Ghirri, P. Neonatal screening for congenital cytomegalovirus infection in preterm and small for gestational age infants. *J. Matern.-Fetal Neonatal Med.* **2014**, *27*, 1589–1593. [CrossRef] [PubMed]

63. Dar, L.; Namdeo, D.; Kumar, P.; Thakar, A.; Kant, S.; Rai, S.; Singh, P.K.; Kabra, M.; Fowler, K.B.; Boppana, S.B. Congenital Cytomegalovirus Infection and Permanent Hearing Loss in Rural North Indian Children. *Pediatr. Infect. Dis. J.* **2017**, *36*, 670–673. [CrossRef] [PubMed]
64. Lin, C.; Tomio, J.; Tanaka, H.; Sonoda, M.; Sano, K.; Kobayashi, Y. Diagnosis and medical care for congenital cytomegalovirus infection: An observational study using claims data in Japan, 2010 to 2017. *Medicine* **2020**, *99*, e19419. [CrossRef]
65. Riga, M.; Korres, G.; Chouridis, P.; Naxakis, S.; Danielides, V. Congenital cytomegalovirus infection inducing non-congenital sensorineural hearing loss during childhood; a systematic review. *Int. J. Pediatr. Otorhinolaryngol.* **2018**, *115*, 156–164. [CrossRef]
66. Kummer, P.; Marcrum, S.C. Potential Benefit of Selective CMV Testing after Failed Newborn Hearing Screening. *Int. J. Neonatal Screen.* **2018**, *4*, 20. [CrossRef]
67. Ronchi, A.; Shimamura, M.; Malhotra, P.S.; Sánchez, P.J. Encouraging postnatal cytomegalovirus (CMV) screening: The time is NOW for universal screening! *Expert Rev. Anti-Infect. Ther.* **2017**, *15*, 417–419. [CrossRef]
68. Kadambari, S.; Luck, S.; Davis, A.; Walter, S.; Agrup, C.; Atkinson, C.; Stimson, L.; Williams, E.; Berrington, J.; Griffiths, P.; et al. Evaluating the feasibility of integrating salivary testing for congenital CMV into the Newborn Hearing Screening Programme in the UK. *Eur. J. Pediatr.* **2015**, *174*, 1117–1121. [CrossRef]

children

MDPI

Review

The Otoacoustic Emissions in the Universal Neonatal Hearing Screening: A Scoping Review Update on the African Data (2004 to 2024)

Stavros Hatzopoulos [1], Ludovica Cardinali [2], Piotr Henryk Skarzynski [3,4,5] and Giovanna Zimatore [6,*]

1. Clinic of Audiology & ENT, University of Ferrara, 44121 Ferrara, Italy; sdh1@unife.it
2. Department of Life Science, Health, and Health Professions, Link Campus University, 00165 Rome, Italy; l.cardinali@unilink.it
3. Heart Failure and Cardiac Rehabilitation Department, Faculty of Medicine and Dentistry, Medical University of Warsaw, 02-005 Warsaw, Poland; piotrhskarzynski@gmail.com
4. Institute of Sensory Organs, 05-830 Kajetany, Poland
5. World Hearing Center, Department of Teleaudiology and Screening, Institute of Physiology and Pathology of Hearing, 02-042 Warsaw, Poland
6. Department of Theoretical and Applied Sciences Applied Physics, eCampus University, 22060 Novedrate, Italy

* Correspondence: giovanna.zimatore@uniecampus.it

Abstract: Background: The reported data on African universal neonatal hearing screening (UNHS) practices tend to be quite scarce, despite the developments in hearing screening the last two decades. The objective of this systematic review was (a) to identify the most recent (in a 20-year span) literature information about NHS/UNHS programs in Africa and (b) to provide data on the procedures used to assess the population, the intervention policies, and on the estimated prevalence of congenital hearing loss with an emphasis on bilateral hearing loss cases. **Methods**: Queries were conducted via the PubMed, Scopus, and Google Scholar databases for the time window of 2004–2024. The mesh terms used were "OAE", "universal neonatal hearing screening", "congenital hearing loss", "well babies", and "Africa". Only research articles and review papers were considered as good candidates. The standard English language filter was not used, to identify information from non-English-speaking scientific communities and groups. **Results**: Data from 15 papers were considered, reflecting the neonatal hearing practices of nine African states. No country-wide NHS programs were reported. The various screening realities are implemented within big urban centers, leaving the residents of rural areas unassisted. For the latter, proposals based on tele-medicine protocols have been suggested. The data on HL prevalence are also incomplete, but the available data refer to rates from 3 to 360 subjects per 1000. These data cannot be taken at face value but within the small sample size context in which they were acquired. Regarding the causes of HL, very few data have been reported; consanguinity is the most attributed factor, at least in the Sub-Saharan African states. For the majority of the programs, no data were reported on hearing loss prevalence/incidence or on any strategies to restore hearing. **Conclusions**: The information on the African neonatal hearing screening are quite scarce, and it is an urgent need to convince audiologists from the African localized programs to publish their hearing screening data.

Keywords: congenital hearing loss; newborn hearing screening; otoacoustic emissions; well babies; NICU; bilateral hearing loss

https://doi.org/10.3390/children12020141

1. Introduction

Neonatal hearing screening (NHS) is an early hearing detection and intervention strategy, which aims to identify infants with potential conductive and sensorineural hearing deficits. Data in the literature strongly suggest that the early detection and rehabilitation of a hearing impairment are essential factors for the development of language and the relative social and cognitive skills [1,2]. At present, two clinical methodologies are available to conduct universal neonatal hearing screening (UNHS); these protocols are based on otoacoustic emissions (OAEs) or on automated auditory brainstem responses (AABR) [3,4]. The basic details on the impact of hearing screening to language development and the inner workings of the clinical screening protocols have been presented in a previous paper [5].

OAEs are a quick, non-invasive, and cost-effective technique. A tiny probe is inserted into the newborn's ear canal, and its microphones produce certain transient stimuli (such as clicks, chirps, and tone busts). A short period of time, measured in milliseconds, is then recorded by the same microphones, which capture the acoustical echoes produced by the inner ear reflecting the stimulus energy [5]. This sort of technology has wide-ranging applications, extending to the detection of age-related hearing loss in adults [6] and in noise-induced hearing loss [7], where a new proposed protocol can identify hearing impairment much earlier than the conventional pure-tone audiometry and the classical TEOAE pass/fail screening criteria.

Even though hearing screening is considered an established clinical practice, NHS programs seem to face many implementation difficulties, as we have previously shown in a review of the European NHS data [5]. Extrapolating this information to states where economic and cultural difficulties are very present (i.e., the stigma related to a hearing loss) [8] is a challenge. Africa is a continent with numerous developing economies, and NHS information is seriously lacking in the literature. As early as 2008, Swanepoel and Storbeck [9] provided initial information on the UNHS-EDHI (early detection and hearing intervention) practices in Africa, with more emphasis in the activities of South Africa. Nevertheless, sixteen years later, Yoshinaga-Itano [10] reported that we still face a lack of screening outcome data (i.e., intervention policies) from African UNHS programs. That statement drove the impetus to discover all possible information about the hearing screening practices in African countries and summarize them within a scoping review.

In addition, the paper has sought suitable responses (when information was attainable from the literature) to the following five issues which are very fundamental for the EDHI strategies: (i) Which countries perform NHS/UNHS? (ii) What percentage of newborns are involved? (iii) How many present congenital deafness and more precisely bilateral deafness? (iv) What is the follow-up rate? (v) Which are the most common protocols and OAE technologies used to assess hearing?

2. Materials and Methods

We sourced scientific articles and reviews using the PubMed, Scopus, and Google Scholar search engines. As in the previous review on the NHS practices in Europe, we have selected a search time-span window of the last 20 years. The main reason for selecting this time window is that the majority of the centralized NHS screening programs [1,10] appear after the year 2000, aided by the fact that the screening technology became quite affordable, with the appearance in the market of portable automated OAE (AOAE) and AABR screeners.

The African continent is composed by 54 countries. In various contexts, Africa is being divided into the northern part and the Sub-Saharan part, which includes 50 states. In this review, we have considered the whole continent without any specific geographical divisions. We focused our investigation on the 84.45% of the total African population (1,532,073,577 as measured in 2024 and reported in [11]), in terms of the first 25 population-dense African states, which are shown in Table 1.

Table 1. Assessed countries for the presence NHS activities. The cells in gray indicate the countries where hearing screening data have been published.

ID	Country	Population	Region	Screening Program
1	Nigeria	232,679,478	Western Africa	Partial
2	Ethiopia	132,059,767	Eastern Africa	Partial
3	Egypt	116,538,258	Northern Africa	Partial
4	DR Congo	109,276,265	Middle Africa	none
5	Tanzania	68,560,157	Eastern Africa	none
6	South Africa	64,007,187	Southern Africa	Partial
7	Kenya	56,432944	Eastern Africa	Partial
8	Sudan	50,448,963	Northern Africa	none
9	Uganda	50,015,092	Eastern Africa	Partial
10	Algeria	46,814,308	Northern Africa	none
11	Morocco	38,081,173	Northern Africa	none
12	Angola	37,885,849	Middle Africa	none
13	Mozambique	34,631,766	Eastern Africa	none
14	Ghana	34,427,414	Western Africa	Partial
15	Madagascar	31,964,956	Eastern Africa	none
16	Côte d'Ivoire	31,934,230	Western Africa	Partial
17	Cameroon	29,123,744	Middle Africa	none
18	Niger	27,032,412	Western Africa	none
19	Mali	24,478,595	Western Africa	none
20	Burkina Faso	23,548,781	Western Africa	none
21	Malawi	21,655,286	Eastern Africa	none
22	Zambia	21,314,956	Eastern Africa	none
23	Chad	20,299,123	Middle Africa	none
24	Somalia	19,009,151	Eastern Africa	none
25	Senegal	18,501,984	Western Arica	none

The literature search, conducted on November 2024, followed the PRISMA 2020 guidelines (the PRISMA website was visited in July 2024, see Table S1) and utilized the following 5 keywords and phrases (mesh terms): "OAE", "neonatal hearing screening", "congenital hearing loss", "well babies" and "Africa". Only research articles and review papers were considered as good candidates. The standard English language filter was not used, to identify possible information from non-English-speaking (i.e., French) scientific communities and groups. Papers related to NHS practices outside the African continent were not considered.

The quality of the material was dictated by several factors, with the publication being in a peer review journal being the cardinal one. Additionally, clearly stated methodologies and a rigorous application of the established screening protocols were also taken into consideration.

The selection criteria for the candidates of the search were based on (i) the origin of the paper (African group or not); (ii) the number of infants screened (large sample studies were preferred), and (iii) the most recent data per country (the most recent study/studies per country were selected).

The surprising fact about the lack of European screening data, we have previously reported in [5], was also repeated for the African countries. Therefore, the stringent criteria we had apply for the European states were lessened. Due to lack of information, we decided to include local studies even referring to small samples, to obtain a glimpse of the screening characteristics of the assessed population.

The PubMed, Scopus, and Google Scholar bibliographic data were considered. Two independent reviewers went over the available material (74 manuscripts), and the final number of eligible papers were distilled to 15 (related to 9 NHS realities, not UNHS, programs). The papers included a thesis dedicated to the status of NHS in the Sub-Saharan area.

The PRISMA flowchart process is reported in Figure 1, and the suitable papers for review are reported in Table 2.

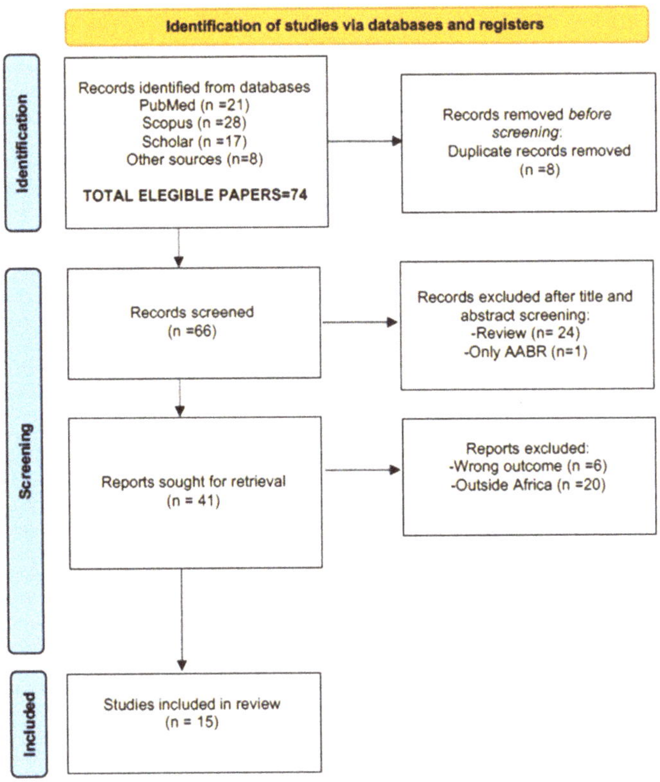

Figure 1. Flow diagram of literature search, according to PRISMA criteria (http://www.prisma-statement.org/, accessed 30 July 2024), with the steps followed in the manuscript selection procedure. After the application of the selection criteria, the initial 74 manuscripts were reduced to 15. Note: the "wrong outcome" voice implies that certain manuscripts were erroneously selected, for example providing data on onchocerciasis-associated epilepsy (OAE) and not on otoacoustic emissions.

Table 2. The 15 eligible papers after the filtering process. The national data are presented in alphabetical order. NA% implies that the data for the population coverage were not available (as in the case of isolated local studies).

n	Country	Sample Size (n)	Year the Study Was Carried Out, Population % Coverage	Authors	Publication Year
1	Cameroon	NA	NA%	Tingang et al.	2020
2	Cote d'Ivoire	Pilot study 1495	July 2007 to March 2008 NA%	Tanon-Anoh et al.	2009
3	Egypt	150	2009 and March 2010 NA%	Imam et al.	2013
4	Ghana	50	NA, NA%	Ameyaw et al.	2019

Table 2. *Cont.*

n	Country	Sample Size (n)	Year the Study Was Carried Out, Population % Coverage	Authors	Publication Year
5	Kenya	9963	NA, NA%	Ndegwa et al.	2024
6	Nigeria	1745	July 2005 to December 2006, NA%	Olusanya et al.	2009
7		4718	NA, NA%	Olusanya et al.	2010
8	Sudan	1120	Feb 2014 to Feb 2019 NA%	Kardman et al.	2023
9	South Africa	510	5 months, NA%	Swanepoel et al.	2006
10		6241	4 y, NA%	Swanepoel et al.	2007
11		32	NA%	Storbeck and Pittman	2008
12		490	NA, NA%	Bezuidenhout et al.	2018
13	Uganda	401	NA, NA%	Seguya et al.	2021
14		1217	NA, NA%	Ndoleriire et al.	2022
15	Sub-Saharan area	NA	NA, NA%	Engelman	2014

3. Results

The data were classified alphabetically, according to the country of origin, and the obtained information is summarized in Table 3, at the end of this section. Figure 2 depicts the African countries where NHS practices are reported.

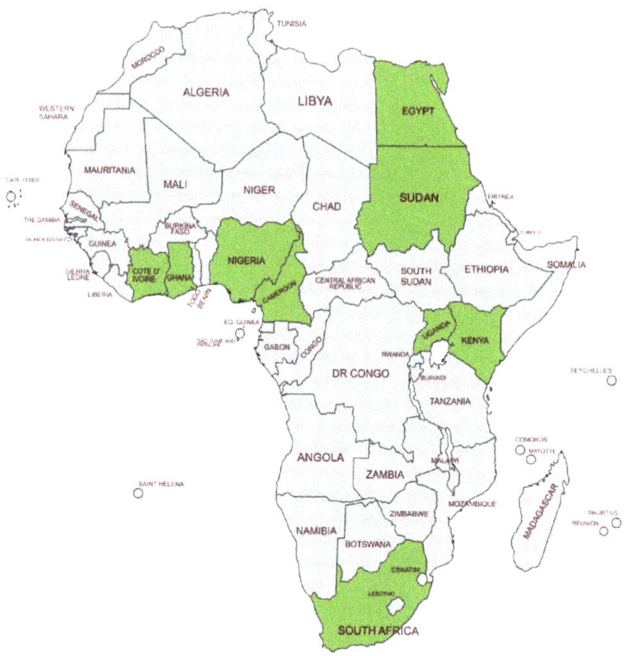

Figure 2. Political map of Africa showing the countries, in green, where NHS activities have been reported in the literature. These African states are reported alphabetically in Table 2.

3.1. Cameroon

There are no NHS data from Cameroon, but there is information on the hearing impairment status across various strata of the Cameroon society. Tingang et al. [12] report that the prevalence of hearing impairment (HI) in Cameroon ranges from 0.9% to 3.6% in population-based studies and increases with age. Environmental factors contribute to 52.6% to 62.2% of HI cases, with meningitis, impacted wax, and age-related disorders being the most common ones. Hereditary HI comprises 0.8% to 14.8% of all cases. In 32.6% to 37% of HI cases, the origin remains unknown. Non-syndromic hearing impairment (NSHI) is the most frequent clinical entity and accounts for 86.1% to 92.5% of cases of HI of genetic origin. Waardenburg and Usher syndromes account for 50% to 57.14% and 8.9% to 42.9% of genetic syndromic cases, respectively. No pathogenic mutation was described in the GJB6 gene, and the prevalence of pathogenic mutations in GJB2 gene ranged from 0% to 0.5%.

The prevalence of permanent hearing loss in Cameroon was found to be from 0.9% to 3.6% (9–36 per 1000), increasing with age.

3.2. Cote d'Ivoire

There is only one pilot study on this country dating back to 2009, which was conducted by Tanon-Anoh et al. [13] at the Abidjan, which is the economic capital of the country. The authors tested well babies (WB) and neonatal intensive care unit (NICU) residents (from 3 to 28 days), simulating a UNHS program. The testing protocol consisted by of a double TEOAE test in the first phase and clinical ABR, tympanometry, and OAEs in the second phase.

They reported the following: "1306 newborns, of a total of 1495, were successfully screened, giving a screening coverage of 87.4%. The average age was 4.5 days, with 5.85 days for the immunization group and 3.20 days for the neonatal unit group. After the second-stage screening, 48 (16.8%) were scheduled for diagnostic evaluation (45 from NICU and 3 from primary care centers). The overall referral rate for diagnostic evaluation was 3.7% (48/1306). Only 18.75% of those referred (9/48) returned for evaluation, and seven of them (77.8%) were confirmed with hearing loss".

The prevalence of permanent hearing loss in this screened population was 5.96 per 1000 (7/1174 babies who completed the screening).

3.3. Egypt

There is no UNHS or NHS program in Egypt. The only information from the Egyptian hearing screening comes from the publication by Imam et al. [14] on the evaluation of targeted versus universal screening practices. The authors employed a rather small sample of 150 infants, including 50 well babies and 100 NICU residents. The NICU residents were divided into two groups: one with only one risk factor (50 infants) termed low risk and one presenting 3–4 risk factors (50 infants) termed high-risk. The testing protocol consisted by of a double TEOAE test in the first phase and clinical ABR, tympanometry, and OAEs in the second phase. Their findings support that a UNHS approach to screening is preferable to a targeted one.

Analytically, the authors report the following: "The most frequent risk factor was consanguinity (46%). In the well-baby population, 16% failed TEOAEs. In the NICU, 30% of the low risk and 38% of the high-risk groups failed TEOAEs. Regarding ABR, failed results were 12%, 10%, and 8% in the high-risk, low-risk, and healthy groups, respectively. Conclusion. The use of targeted screening would have missed 8% of neonates from the well-baby group who present permanent congenital hearing loss".

The authors also speculate on the high estimates of the hearing impairment encountered in their sample, referring to other analyses, which have supported the presence of connexin 26 (Cx26) mutations and alterations in the southern Egyptian population [15].

Due to the small sample used in the study, the estimated incidence of hearing loss of 360 per 1000 is obviously erroneous, as it was based on selected cases and not on a rather large and randomized sample.

3.4. Ghana

According Ameyaw et al. [16], in Ghana, there is an established infant hearing screening, as part of its Early Hearing Detection and Intervention program. However, because of the lack of hearing health care specialists, especially pediatric audiologists, newborn hearing screening and other infant hearing services are accessible only at the Korle-Bu Teaching Hospital (KBTH) located in the Greater Accra Region of Ghana. Data in the literature regarding the EDHI program at KBTH are not available. The paper by Ameyaw et al. describes the results of applying tele-health technologies in neonatal hearing screening. The authors used a sample of 50 infants (aged 2–90 days) in the Brong-Ahafo Regional Hospital. The infants were assessed with a DPOAE protocol from a Bio-Logic AuDX device. The paper is focused on the technical aspects of the tele-health protocol.

Adadey et al. [17], in a paper related to the hearing impairment implications of GJB2 genetic screening in 2020, also report that there is a UNHS program in Ghana that is unavailable in most health centers across the country. For the authors, the failure to effectively establish the UNHS across the country could be due to a variety of reasons, including the high cost of testing, limited infrastructural capacity, and the lack of human resources to man the service.

3.5. Kenya

There is no NHS or UNHS running program in Kenya. The most recent data come from the paper of Ndegwa et al. in 2024 [18], describing a pilot UNHS program in the capital city of Nairobi. The authors report the following: "The screening coverage rate was 98.6% (9963/10,104). The referral rate for the initial screen was 3.6% (356/9963), the return rate for follow-up rescreening was 72% (258 babies out of 356) with a Lost To Follow-up rate of 28% (98/356). The referral rate of the second screen was 10% (26/258). All the 26 babies referred from the second screen returned for diagnostic hearing evaluation and were confirmed with hearing loss, yielding a prevalence of 26/9963 = 3 per 1000".

The 26 infants presenting hearing loss were 21 bilateral and 5 unilateral cases. The bilateral cases were composed by four mild, nine moderate, five severe, and three profound hearing loss cases. The paper does not offer any explanation on the causality of the hearing loss, and the authors do not report any intervention policies for the infants presenting hearing loss; although, in their paper, Figure 1 refers to hearing aid fitting after an ENT consultation. Despite the fact the project was funded by MEDEL, no data on any cochlear implant recipients are presented.

3.6. Nigeria

There is no active NHS or UNHS program in Nigeria; although, a number of pilot studies by Olusanya et al. [19,20] have been reported in the literature.

In the first study [19], the authors reported that, of the 3676 infants enrolled, 52.4% were not born in hospital, and 71 (2.1%) were confirmed to have SNHL. For the 13 infants presenting bilateral hearing loss, 3 presented a moderate SNHL, 8 presented a severe SNHL and 3 presented a profound SNHL. One infant presented unilateral loss. Six of the infants with SNHL had a profile suggestive of auditory neuropathy/dys-synchrony. Data on any intervention policies (hearing aids, cochlear implants) are not reported.

The second study [20] was an attempt to evaluate the performance of two major tools in NHS, namely OAEs and AABR. The authors reported that 1745 (36.9%) infants completed both TEOAE and AABR. Of this group, 1060 (60.7%) passed both TEOAE and

AABR ("true-negatives"); 92 (5.3%) failed both TEOAE and AABR ("true-positive"); 571 (32.7%) failed TEOAE but passed AABR ("false-positives"), while 22 (1.3%) passed TEOAE but failed AABR ("false-negatives"). No HL incidence is reported.

3.7. Sudan

There is no NHS or UNHS program in Sudan, and the only hearing screening report available is a paper from Kardman et al. [21], in 2023, on a project conducted in the capital of the country Khartoum. The authors assessed 736 NICU residents and 384 well babies over a period of 5 years, using TEOAEs and a clinical ABR. From the risk factors reported, consanguinity, ototoxic drugs, gestational age, and neonatal jaundice were the most reported. From the NICU infants, 16 did not pass the TEOAE screening test, and the authors reported some problems with 8 NICU infants who were scheduled to be retested. Only 8 infants were evaluated with an ABR and all presented bilateral hearing loss. The estimated prevalence in this group was reported as 10.8 per 1000, which is underestimated, since 50% of the referred subjects were not assessed by ABR. From the 384 well babies, 6 failed the TEOAE test. From those, four did not return for the clinical ABR, and the other two were verified with SNHL. The HL incidence of the well-baby group was reported as 5.2 per 1000, which is also an underestimate of the true incidence, since 66.6% of the referred infants were not assessed with ABR.

3.8. South Africa

According to Bezuidenhout et al. [22], the state of South Africa is the most developed in terms of hearing screening practices, but still, no formalized and standardized system of newborn hearing screening (NHS) exists at state-run hospitals in Johannesburg, South Africa (SA). Only risk-based hearing screening occurs, and this is also not systematic. We have identified four manuscripts referring to four different glimpses of NHS development in that country. From the oldest to the newest, these reports are as follows.

The first paper by Swanepoel et al. [23] explored the possibilities to conduct an OAE plus high-frequency tympanometry (1000 Hz) assessment on selected infants, in two private centers for a period of 5 months. The study did not report any HL incidence or any EDHI policies, but the authors reported that "Follow-up screening appointments were scheduled for 68 subjects (14% of screened sample). Only 40% returned for the second follow-up and 44% for the third follow-up".

The second paper by Swanepoel et al. [24] refers to data from a retrospective study on 6241 infants, in a private hospital in urban Gauteng, South Africa. The authors reported that "The overall referral rate for the screening program across the 4 years was 11.1% but referral rates decreased by between 2 and 4% for each year of program existence with a 5% rate in year 4. Only 32% of the rescreens were completed at the hospital, and no data was available for the remaining infants because parents were provided a choice of follow up centers. Referral for a diagnostic assessment after the rescreens at the hospital was predictive of sensorineural hearing loss in one-third of cases and the estimated prevalence was 3 per 1000". Due to the large loss of subjects to be retested by ABR, this value of prevalence underestimates the true HL incidence value in the Gauteng area.

The third paper by Storbeck and Pittman [25] appeared in the 2008 special issue of the International Journal of Audiology, dedicated to the early detection and hearing intervention (EDHI) programs in Africa. The authors reported data "from a family-centred, home-based intervention program (HI HOPES) over a 12-month period in order to track the effectiveness of the holistic unbiased support to families of infants and toddlers with a hearing-loss". The SNHL of the children was classified as "moderate loss 2 cases, moderate to severe loss 4 cases, moderate to profound loss 3 cases, severe to profound loss 7 cases and profound loss 15 cases". For the 32 children who participated in the program, 24 received a digital hearing aid, 3 a cochlear implant; for 1 infant, the family declined amplification, and for another, it was not possible to amplify due to an ear malformation. Obviously, the structure of the project did not permit an estimate of the HL incidence in the assessed areas.

The fourth paper by Bezuidenhoutet al. [22] assessed the challenge of applying a UNHS model in a public context in Johannesburg, South Africa. The project used a double (i.e., test and retest) OAE protocol with TEOAEs or DPOAEs and a clinical ABR for diagnosis. The authors report that "of 2740 neonates born during the study period, 490 (17.9%) were identified for screening, and distortion product otoacoustic emissions screening was conducted on 121 (4.4%). Repeat screening was required in 57 (47.1%) neonates, but only 20 returned for follow-up". The most important challenges to the feasibility of UNHS implementation were the insufficient number of audiologists available to provide screening, the high rate of false positive test results, and the unacceptably high rates of loss to follow-up. Two modifiable factors, namely the presence of vernix caseosa in the external ear canal and high ambient noise levels, were found to have significantly influenced the screening process.

3.9. Uganda

There is no NHS or UNHS in Uganda, and the only information from hearing screening practices comes from two recent papers by Seguya et al. in 2021 [25] and Ndoleriire et al. in 2022 [26]. For both papers, TEOAEs were used for testing and retesting. ABR was used diagnostically in the second phase of the assessment.

In the first paper by Seguya et al., the authors report that "We recruited infants aged 1 day to 3 months and performed a three-staged screening. At stage 1, we used Transient Evoked Oto-acoustic Emissions (TEOAEs), at stage 2 we repeated TEOAEs for infants who failed TEOAEs at stage 1 and at stage 3, we conducted Automated brainstem responses (ABRs) for those who failed stage 2. Infant Hearing Loss (IHL) was present if they failed an ABR at 35 dBHL". A total of 401 infants were tested, and 299 passed stage 1, while the remaining 102 (25.4%) were referred for stage 2. Of those, 35 (34.3%) returned for stage 2 screening. Five infants failed the second TEOAE assessment in at least one ear. From those, four were identified with a unilateral SNHL, and one with a bilateral SNHL. The estimated HL incidence was 14.9 per 1000 (5/334). Unfortunately, this high number is an underestimate of the actual incidence, since only 34.3% of the referred infants returned for the ABR evaluation.

In the second paper by Ndoleriire et al., the authors reported the efficacy of hearing screening in children between 0 and 59 months. The data reported refer to a sample of 1217 children of various ages, tested in two phases with TEOAEs. From those, 27 failed the TEOAE test unilaterally and 18 bilaterally. Factors affecting the TEOAE failure included rural residence ($p = 0.027$), a low birth weight ($p = 0.045$), relatives having hearing loss ($p \leq 0.001$), admission to the hospital after birth ($p = 0.012$), and a history of a childhood suppurative otitis media ($p = 0.015$). No other information on these 45 children is available.

Table 3. Data related to the various African NHS national activities. The national data are presented in alphabetical order. The gray shaded estimates indicate high prevalence values: BD = bilateral deafness; WB = well babies; NICU = infants from the intensive care unit; NA = data not available; HA = hearing aid; CI = cochlear implant.

Country	Participants (n)	Screening Protocol	Hearing Loss Prevalence	Causes	Intervention Policies
Cameroon	NA	NA	9–36 per 1000	Non-syndromic hearing impairment Waardenburg and Usher syndromes	NA
Côte d'Ivoire	1495	TEOAE, clinical ABR	5.96 per 1000	NA	NA
Egypt	150	TEOAE, clinical ABR	360 × 1000	Consanguinity risk factor, presence of I71N mutations in the CJB2 gene	NA
Ghana	50	DPOAE	NA	NA	NA
Kenya	9963	DPOAE + AABR, ABR	3 per 1000	NA	NA
Nigeria	4718		NA	Probable auditory neuropathy in 6/13 SNHL cases	NA
	1745	TEOAE + AABR	NA	NA	NA
Sudan	1120		10.8 per 1000 NICU 5.2 per 1000 WB	NA	NA
South Africa	510	DPOAE + 1000 Hz tymp, ABR	NA	NA	NA
	6241	TEOAE, ABR	3 per 1000	NA	NA
	32	NA	NA		HA (24), CI (3)
	490	TEOAE/DPOAE, ABR	NA	NA	NA
Uganda	401	TEOAE + ABR	14.9 per 1000	NA	NA
	1217	TEOAE + ABR	NA	NA	NA

4. Discussion

The first objective of the paper was to provide updates on the African NHS/UNHS practices, from reports found in the literature in the period 2004–2024. The second objective of the paper was to extract information from the identified ongoing UNHS programs, regarding the coverage of the project, the congenital hearing impairment estimates (with emphasis into the bilateral hearing loss), the description of causes leading to hearing loss and the relative intervention strategies, and lastly, the technologies and protocols used. The sections below summarize the reported data in the assessed 15 manuscripts.

4.1. The Number of NHS Programs

In the previous review on the European NHS-UNHS programs [5], we reported that it was quite surprising to discover that the European data on NHS are very poor, and very few reports exist to describe the actual NHS programs in Europe. The African NHS data in the literature are even more scarce. Of the nine African states where there are reports about an NHS program, none has a functional or presently active cross-country NHS/UNHS. Adadey et al. [17] mentions the existence of a UNHS program in Ghana (from the 1970s), which is not only not active across the whole country, but the output data from screening (i.e., intervention) are unknown. Data from Olusanya [8] and Engelman [27] suggest that, in most African states, there are sporadic local hospital-based screening programs, using the established two-phase OAE assessment with a clinical ABR for third-stage case referrals.

4.2. Reported NHS/UNHS Coverage: Issues of Loss to Follow-Up

There are no data in the literature regarding NHS coverage, in terms of country territories. According to the data in Table 3, most large studies in Kenya [18], Nigeria [20], and South Africa [24] refer to local activities usually spanning a single hospital territory.

An interesting observation of the data in Table 3 is that, in a number of African hearing screening realities [12,17,20,21,25], the percentage level of the loss to follow-up (LTF) infants is quite high (i.e., >15%), especially for subjects who did not pass the first OAE assessment. Generally, the percentage of LTF is an index of the organizing efficiency of the NHS/UNHS program and in European and other Western countries has been initially attributed to loopholes in the NHS phases, i.e., test, retest, etc. [28,29].

More recent studies in the literature have better explored the innerworkings of LTF and have suggested that a number of social and demographic factors have a negative impact on it [30,31]. Factors contributing to a higher LTF include the following: single maternal marital status (the younger the single mothers the higher the LTF), having an insurance policy, the education level of the mother, and the residence of the mother in a rural or in a city location. These factors can be easily identified in any of the African screening realities. In addition, due to lack of extensive parental information [8,22], the social stigma of having hearing loss [32] possibly increases the LTF percentages. The relationship between LTF and social stigma has not been elucidated completely, and additional studies are needed.

4.3. Estimates of Bilateral Hearing Loss Prevalence

The fact that there are no country-wide or large UNHS programs implies that the reported hearing loss incidences are not precise. In many cases, where the authors do not present more detailed data, it is assumed that the reported incidences are an average between NICU infants and well babies.

The highest incidence has been reported in Egypt (360 per 1000) in a rather small sample of selected infants. Other high HL incidences have been reported in Uganda (14.9 per 1000), Sudan (10.8 per 1000 in the NICU), and Cameroon (9–36 per 1000). A note for the latter study using the Cameroon data (Tingtang et al. [11]), the HL prevalence data were assembled not from NHS singular databases but from independent studies in Cameroon, affronting various pathologies that impact hearing.

The studies from both Kenya and Soth Africa (3 per 1000) are closer to the reported norms of European [33] and North American [34] studies and the data released by the World Health Association in 2021, with a prevalence of 3.74 per 1000 [35]. The studies from Kenya and South Africa assessed data from relatively large sample sets (9943 and 6241 cases, respectively), and probably, for this reason, the HL prevalence estimates are closer to the international values. The Nigerian screening reports used large datasets, but unfortunately, the corresponding authors did not provide any HL prevalence data.

4.4. Causes Leading to Hearing Loss and Requiring Intervention Strategies

Data in this section are very scarce, since the majority of the papers have only reported screening performance metrics, rather than the HL prevalence and EDHI strategies.

In terms of risk factors leading to possible HL, data from Egypt [14,15] suggest consanguinity and various mutations of the CJB2 gene. Consanguinity as a risk factor has been reported in other papers from Nigeria [19], South Africa [23], and the Sub-Saharan states [27] and probably mirrors African social practices.

In terms of intervention policies, the literature is extremely vague, and only the paper by Storbeck and Pittman [9] discussed hearing aids and cochlear implants in a group of South African children, within the context of the HI HOPES project.

Considering the lack of screening programs and the presence of only sporadic hearing intervention strategies, it can be assumed that the identification of a hearing deficit and a possible intervention occurs late, probably at early-school age. There are data on this topic; see, for example, Skarzynski et al. [36] on the Lagos schoolchildren screening results and Jesuyajolu et al.'s [37] review on the Nigerian cochlear implant data, but more detailed information in this direction is outside the scope of this review.

4.5. Technological Issues

All the screening papers report data from a two-stage OAE protocol, where the third stage was an AABR or, directly, a diagnostic ABR. Distortion product otoacoustic emissions were used in the papers from Ghana [16], Kenya [18], and South Africa [23]. There is a lack of information on the actual OAE hardware used, but the descriptive information of these projects refers primarily to portable OAE screeners, which probably have the option to carry out an AABR assessment of the tested infant. In this context, no questions were raised regarding the OAE probe calibration issues that we have postulated in previous papers [38,39] and in the European hearing screening data review [5].

4.6. Factors Affecting the NHS Practices in Africa

According to Kanji [36], poor-quality child health services for children who are ill was observed in relation to waiting periods, staff skills, triage, and promotional, prevention, and curative care. This was further accompanied by insufficient developmental assessment. Inconsistency was noticed in terms of immunization and rehabilitation.

Ameyaw et al. [16] pointed out that, because of the lack of hearing healthcare specialists, especially pediatric audiologists, newborn hearing screening and other infant hearing services are accessible only at the Korle-Bu Teaching Hospital (KBTH) located in the Greater Accra Region of Ghana.

Furthermore, Jesuyajolu et al. [37] commented that hearing screening and subsequent interventions in Nigeria are impeded by high cost, lack of full rehabilitative facilities and staff, skepticism, and a lack of funding.

These comments from the clinical realities in South Africa, Ghana, and Nigeria are the background realities of all exposed programs in this review. Economic factors, lack of professional figures, and skepticism related to the stigma of hearing loss are the key players in the resistance to neonatal hearing screening.

Of course, in the last decade, the costs of screening equipment (especially the ones based on OAEs) have decreased significantly, so the key element in the problems listed above is to affront the availability of a professional audiologist. This aspect is much more complicated, because it involves not only educational resources (for the scientific formation of audiology technicians and audiologists) but also a state budget.

One way to address this problem is to develop tele-medicine resources. Various papers in the literature have already addressed not only the feasibility of implementing such a structure in an African reality [16,40–42] but also the possibility of lowering the reported LTF percentages [43]. While the concept of tele-audiology is quite attractive, it should be considered that most of the tele-audiology data come from the state of South Africa. Taking into consideration the economic dimensions of the necessary infrastructure [41], the available data in the literature do not specify whether the tele-audiology model can be exported to all rural African realities, as a solution to a more globalized NHS.

4.7. Limitations of the Study

It might be possible that some publications in local African journals that are not indexed in PubMed or Scopus were not considered in the filtering process of the manuscript evaluation. On the other hand, such manuscripts (with no impact factor) would challenge the quality criteria we have imposed on this scoping review.

4.8. Future Directions

More clinical studies are required to identify and assess the cultural attitudes toward hearing loss and how stigma might influence screening acceptance and follow-up. There is also a need for more information regarding the transition from NHS to EDHI.

This last section was requested by one of the reviewers of the manuscript who posed the interesting question of whether an improvement of hearing screening practices in Africa could generally improve the audiological services to those in need. Theoretically, the answer should have been a "yes". However, the available data from the African screening policies do not support such a relationship for at least two main reasons, as follows: (1) the level of the audiological services depends heavily on the local economics [28,37] and (2) the availability or rather the lack of audiology professionals per territory [8,16]. The data presented also suggest that the social stigma of deafness and the lack of extensive information to the families [40] might worsen the synergy between an NHS program and other audiological intervention services, causing high levels of loss to follow-up (LFU), discussed in Section 4.2.

In summary, the lack of precise hearing screening and follow-up data results in a lack of a workable model exploring the effects of a successful NHS program on the general audiological services. This sort of information needs to be elucidated as soon as possible.

5. Conclusions

The data on the African neonatal hearing screening are quite scarce, and no country-wise programs exist at the moment. The various screening realities are implemented within big urban centers, leaving the residents of rural areas unassisted. For the latter, proposals based on tele-medicine protocols have been suggested.

The data on HL prevalence are also incomplete, but the available data refer to rates from 3 to 360 subjects per 1000. These data cannot be taken at face value but within the small-sample size context in which they were acquired.

Regarding the causes of HL, very few data have reported that consanguinity is the most attributed factor, at least in the Sub-Saharan African states.

Supplementary Materials: The following supporting information can be downloaded at: https://www.mdpi.com/article/10.3390/children12020141/s1, Table S1: PRISMA 2020 Checklist [44].

Author Contributions: Bibliographic search, S.H., G.Z. and L.C., investigation, data curation: S.H., G.Z. and L.C.; writing—original draft preparation, S.H. and G.Z.; writing—review and editing, S.H., G.Z. and P.H.S. All authors have read and agreed to the published version of the manuscript.

Funding: This research received no external funding.

Institutional Review Board Statement: Not applicable.

Informed Consent Statement: Not applicable.

Data Availability Statement: Data available upon request.

Conflicts of Interest: The authors declare no conflicts of interest.

Abbreviations

AABR	Automated auditory brainstem response
ABR	Auditory brainstem response
BD	Bilateral deafness
EDHI	Early hearing detection and intervention
NICU	Neonatal intensive care unit
OAE	Otoacoustic emissions
UNHS	Universal neonatal hearing screening

References

1. Yoshinaga-Itano, C. Benefits of early intervention for Children with Hearing Loss. *Otolaryngol. Clin. N. Am.* **1999**, *32*, 1089–1102. [CrossRef]
2. Downs, M.P.; Yoshinaga-Itano, C. The Efficacy of early identification and intervention in children with hearing impairment. *Pediatr. Clin. N. Am.* **1999**, *46*, 79–87. [CrossRef]
3. Kemp, D.T. Stimulated acoustic emissions from within the human auditory system. *J. Acoust. Soc. Am.* **1978**, *64*, 1386–1391. [CrossRef] [PubMed]
4. Mason, J.A.; Hermann, K.R. Universal infant hearing screening by automated auditory brainstem response measurement. *Pediatrics* **1998**, *101*, 221–228. [CrossRef] [PubMed]
5. Hatzopoulos, S.; Cardinali, L.; Skarżyński, P.H.; Zimatore, G. The Otoacoustic Emissions in the Universal Neonatal Hearing Screening: An Update on the European Data (2004 to 2024). *Children* **2024**, *11*, 1276. [CrossRef]
6. Zimatore, G.; Cavagnaro, M.; Skarzynski, P.H.; Fetoni, A.R.; Hatzopoulos, S. Detection of age-related hearing losses (Arhl) via transient-evoked otoacoustic emissions. *Clin. Interv. Aging* **2020**, *15*, 927–935. [CrossRef] [PubMed]
7. Zimatore, G.; Fetoni, A.R.; Paludetti, G.; Cavagnaro, M.; Podda, M.V.; Troiani, D. Post-processing analysis of transient-evoked otoacoustic emissions to detect 4 kHz-notch hearing impairment—A pilot study (2011). *Med. Sci. Monit.* **2011**, *17*, MT41–MT49. [CrossRef]
8. Olusanya, B.O. Priorities for early hearing detection and intervention in sub-Saharan Africa. *Int. J. Audiol.* **2008**, *47* (Suppl. S1), S3–S13. [CrossRef] [PubMed]
9. Swanepoel, D.; Störbeck, C. EHDI Africa: Advocating for infants with hearing loss in Africa. *Int. J. Audiol.* **2008**, *47* (Suppl. S1), S1–S2. [CrossRef]
10. Yoshinaga-Itano, C.; Carr, G.; Davis, A.; Ching, T.Y.C.; Chung, K.; Clark, J.; Harkus, S.; Kuan, M.-L.; Garg, S.; Balen, S.A.; et al. Coalition for Global Hearing Health Hearing Care Pathways Working Group: Guidelines for Clinical Guidance for Readiness and Development of Evidence-Based Early Hearing Detection and Intervention Programs. *Ear Hear.* **2024**, *45*, 1071–1088. [CrossRef] [PubMed]
11. Worlmeter Website. Available online: https://www.worldometers.info/world-population/africa-population/ (accessed on 15 December 2024).

12. Tingang, E.W.; Noubiap, J.J.; Fokouo, J.V.F.; Oluwole, O.G.; Nguefack, S.; Chimusa, E.R.; Wonkam, A. Hearing Impairment Overview in Africa: The Case of Cameroon. *Genes* **2020**, *11*, 233. [CrossRef] [PubMed]
13. Tanon-Anoh, M.; Sanogo-Gone, D.; Kouassi, K. Newborn Hearing Screening in a Developing Country: Results of a Pilot Study in Abidjan, Côte D'ivoire. *Int. J. Pediatr. Otorhinolaryngol.* **2010**, *74*, 188–191. [CrossRef] [PubMed]
14. Imam, S.S.; El-Farrash, R.A.; Taha, H.M.; Bishoy, H.E. Targeted versus Universal Neonatal Hearing Screening in a Single Egyptian Center. *Int. Sch. Res. Not.* **2013**, *2013*, 574937. [CrossRef]
15. Mohamed, M.R.; Alesutan, I.; Föller, M.; Sopjani, M.; Bress, A.; Baur, M.; Salama, R.H.; Bakr, M.S.; Mohamed, M.A.; Blin, N.; et al. Functional Analysis of a Novel I71N Mutation in the GJB2 Gene among Southern Egyptians Causing Autosomal Recessive Hearing Loss. *Cell. Physiol. Biochem.* **2010**, *26*, 959–966. [CrossRef] [PubMed]
16. Ameyaw, G.A.; Ribera, J.; Anim-Sampong, S. Interregional Newborn Hearing Screening via Telehealth in Ghana. *J. Am. Acad. Audiol.* **2019**, *30*, 178–186. [CrossRef] [PubMed]
17. Adadey, S.M.; Quaye, O.; Amedofu, G.K.; Awandare, G.A.; Wonkam, A. Screening for GJB2-R143W-Associated Hearing Impairment: Implications for Health Policy and Practice in Ghana. *Public Health Genom.* **2020**, *23*, 184–189. [CrossRef] [PubMed]
18. Ndegwa, S.; Tucci, D.; Lemons, J.; Murila, F.; Shepherd, S.; Mwangi, M.; Macharia, I.; Ayugi, J. Newborn and Infant Hearing Screening for Early Detection of Hearing Loss in Nairobi, Kenya. *Afr. Health Sci.* **2024**, *24*, 228–238. [CrossRef] [PubMed]
19. Olusanya, B.O.; Somefun, A.O. Sensorineural Hearing Loss in Infants with Neonatal Jaundice in Lagos: A Community-Based Study. *Ann. Trop. Paediatr.* **2009**, *29*, 119–128. [CrossRef] [PubMed]
20. Olusanya, B.O.; Bamigboye, B.A. Is Discordance in TEOAE and AABR Outcomes Predictable in Newborns? *Int. J. Pediatr. Otorhinolaryngol.* **2010**, *74*, 1303–1309. [CrossRef] [PubMed]
21. Kardman, S.E.; Omer, E.M.; Abdalla, N.; Khalid, M.; Kheir, M. Neonatal hearing screening in Soba University Hospital, Khartoum, Sudan: A cross-sectional study. *Egypt. J. Otolaryngol.* **2023**, *39*, 2. [CrossRef]
22. Bezuidenhout, J.K.; Khoza-Shangase, K.; De Maayer, T.; Strehlau, R. Universal newborn hearing screening in public healthcare in South Africa: Challenges to implementation. *S. Afr. J. Child. Health* **2018**, *12*, 159–163. [CrossRef]
23. Swanepoel, D.W.; Hugo, R.; Louw, B. Infant hearing screening at immunization clinics in South Africa. *Int. J. Pediatr. Otorhinolaryngol.* **2006**, *70*, 1241–1249. [CrossRef] [PubMed]
24. Swanepoel, D.; Ebrahim, S.; Joseph, A.; Friedland, P.L. Newborn hearing screening in a South African private health care hospital. *Int. J. Pediatr. Otorhinolaryngol.* **2007**, *71*, 881–887. [CrossRef] [PubMed]
25. Störbeck, C.; Pittman, P. Early Intervention in South Africa: Moving beyond Hearing Screening. *Int. J. Audiol.* **2008**, *47* (Suppl. S1), S36–S43. [CrossRef] [PubMed]
26. Seguya, A.; Bajunirwe, F.; Kakande, E.; Nakku, D. Feasibility of Establishing an Infant Hearing Screening Program and Measuring Hearing Loss among Infants at a Regional Referral Hospital in South Western Uganda. *PLoS ONE* **2021**, *16*, e0253305. [CrossRef]
27. Ndoleriire, C.; Ssenyonjo, K.D.; Fiona, K.; Bisso, F.; Nakku, D.; Okema, L.; Mukiibi, I.; Nakafeero, M.; Nyabigambo, A.; Matsiko, S.; et al. Implementing Hearing Screening among Children Aged 0–59 Months at Established Immunization Clinics in Uganda: A Multi-Center Study. *Int. J. Pediatr. Otorhinolaryngol.* **2023**, *164*, 111397. [CrossRef] [PubMed]
28. Engelman, D. The Status of Neonatal Hearing Screening in Sub-Saharan Africa. A Systematic Review. Ph.D. Thesis, City University of New York, New York, NY, USA, 2014.
29. Raynor, E.; Holmes, C.; Crowson, M.; Peskoe, S.; Planey, A.; Lantos, P.M. Loss to follow up of failed hearing screen and missed opportunities to detect congenital cytomegalovirus are better identified with the implementation of a new electronic health record system protocol. *Int. J. Pediatr. Otorhinolaryngol.* **2021**, *148*, 110818. [CrossRef]
30. Cunningham, M.; Thomson, V.; McKiever, E.; Dickinson, L.M.; Furniss, A.; Allison, M.A. Infant, maternal, and hospital factors' role in loss to follow-up after failed newborn hearing screening. *Acad. Pediatr.* **2018**, *18*, 188–195. [CrossRef] [PubMed]
31. Atherton, K.M.; Poupore, N.S.; Clemmens, C.S.; Nietert, P.J.; Pecha, P.P. Sociodemographic Factors Affecting Loss to Follow-Up After Newborn Hearing Screening: A Systematic Review and Metaanalysis. *Otolaryngol. Head Neck Surg.* **2023**, *168*, 1289–1300. [CrossRef] [PubMed]
32. Best, K.C.; Ameh, E.; Weldon, C.; Shwe, D.; Maigari, I.M.; Turaki, I.; Shehu, N.Y. Double stigma: A cross-sectional study of Lassa patients with hearing loss in North Central Nigeria. *Front. Public Health* **2024**, *12*, 1395939. [CrossRef] [PubMed]
33. Erixon, E. Estimated prevalence of permanent hearing loss among newborns and 6-year-olds: An evaluation of the three auditory screenings in Uppsala. *Int. J. Pediatr. Otorhinolaryngol.* **2024**, *176*, 111785. [CrossRef] [PubMed]
34. Dundon, K.; Ema, S.; Deng, X.; Morrison, M.; Brown, T.; White, K.; Hazard, L.; Fort, M.; Coverstone, K.; Mason, C.A.; et al. Likely Impact of the COVID-19 Pandemic on Newborn Hearing Screening and Follow-up Services in the United States in 2020. *J. Early Hear. Detect. Interv.* **2022**, *7*, 1–5. [CrossRef]
35. World Health Organization. World Report on Hearing. 2021. Available online: https://www.who.int/publications/i/item/9789240020481 (accessed on 17 December 2024).
36. Skarzynski, P.H.; Swierniak, W.; Gos, E.; Bienkowska, K.; Adeyinka, P.; Olubi, O.; Afolabi, S.; Skarzynska, M.B.; Hatzopoulos, S. Pilot Hearing Screening of School-age Children in Lagos, Nigeria. *J. Health Care Poor Underserved* **2021**, *32*, 1444–1460. [CrossRef] [PubMed]

37. Jesuyajolu, D.; Obuh, O.; Edeh, E. Overcoming Developing-World Challenges in Cochlear Implantation: A Nigerian Perspective. *Ann. Med. Surg.* **2023**, *85*, 5533–5537. [CrossRef] [PubMed]
38. Zimatore, G.; Skarzynski, P.H.; Di Berardino, F.; Filipponi, E.; Hatzopoulos, S. Differences between pressurized and non-pressurized transient-evoked otoacoustic emissions in neonatal subjects. *Audiol. Neurotol.* **2021**, *26*, 346–352. [CrossRef]
39. Zimatore, G.; Skarzynski, P.H.; Di Berardino, F.; Gasbarre, A.M.; Filipponi, E.; Araimo, G.; Hatzopoulos, S. Re-evaluating the scoring criteria of the Interacoustics Sera Neonatal Hearing Screener. *Hear. Balance Commun.* **2024**, *22*, 100–109. [CrossRef]
40. Kanji, A. Newborn and infant hearing screening at primary healthcare clinics in South Africa designated as National Health Insurance pilot sites: An exploratory study. *S. Afr. J. Commun. Disord.* **2022**, *69*, 7. [CrossRef]
41. Bhutta, M.F.; Swanepoel, D.W.; Fagan, J. ENT from Afar: Opportunities for Remote Patient Assessment, Clinical Management, Teaching and Learning. *Clin. Otolaryngol.* **2021**, *46*, 689–691. [CrossRef] [PubMed]
42. Frisby, C.; Eikelboom, R.; Mahomed-Asmail, F.; Kuper, H.; Swanepoel, D.W. M-Health Applications for Hearing Loss: A Scoping Review. *Telemed. E-Health* **2022**, *28*, 1090–1099. [CrossRef] [PubMed]
43. Dharmar, M.; Simon, A.; Sadorra, C.; Friedland, G.; Sherwood, J.; Morrow, H.; Deines, D.; Nickell, D.; Lucatorta, D.; Marcin, J.P. Reducing loss to follow-up with tele-audiology diagnostic evaluations. *Telemed. J. E Health* **2016**, *22*, 159–164. [CrossRef] [PubMed]
44. Page, M.J.; McKenzie, J.E.; Bossuyt, P.M.; Boutron, I.; Hoffmann, T.C.; Mulrow, C.D.; Shamseer, L.; Tetzlaff, J.M.; Akl, E.A.; Brennan, S.E.; et al. The PRISMA 2020 statement: An updated guideline for reporting systematic reviews. *BMJ* **2021**, *372*, n71. [CrossRef] [PubMed]

children

MDPI

Systematic Review

Systematic Review on Microtia: Current Knowledge and Future Directions

Filippo Hellies [1,†], Silvia Fracaro [1,†], Gino Marioni [2], Annalisa Trotta [1], Martina Todesco [3], Martina Casarin [4], Andrea Bagno [3], Elisabetta Zanoletti [5], Giovanna Albertin [6] and Laura Astolfi [1,*]

1 Bioacoustics Research Laboratory, Department of Neuroscience-DNS, University of Padova, 35128 Padova, Italy; filippo.hellies@phd.unipd.it (F.H.); silvia.fracaro@phd.unipd.it (S.F.); annalisa.trotta@studenti.univr.it (A.T.)
2 Phoniatrics and Audiology Unit, Department of Neuroscience-DNS, University of Padova, 31100 Treviso, Italy; gino.marioni@unipd.it
3 Department of Industrial Engineering, University of Padova, Via Marzolo 9, 35131 Padova, Italy; martina.todesco.2@phd.unipd.it (M.T.); andrea.bagno@unipd.it (A.B.)
4 Department of Surgery, Oncology and Gastroenterology, University of Padova, Giustiniani 2, 35128 Padova, Italy; martina.casarin@unipd.it
5 Section of Otorhinolaryngology-Head and Neck Surgery, Department of Neuroscience-DNS, "Azienda Ospedale Università di Padova"-University of Padova, 35128 Padova, Italy; elisabetta.zanoletti@unipd.it
6 Section of Human Anatomy, Department of Neuroscience-DNS, University of Padova, Via Gabelli 65, 35122 Padova, Italy; giovanna.albertin@unipd.it
* Correspondence: laura.astolfi@unipd.it; Tel.: +39-0498217452
† These authors contributed equally to this work.

Abstract: Background: Microtia is a congenital outer ear deformity that causes the auricle to be absent or underdeveloped. It is frequently associated with external auditory canal atresia and causes hearing and psychosocial problems. Objectives: We thoroughly investigate the aspects of microtia and explore both current and innovative therapies. Methods: A systematic literature review was conducted following PRISMA guidelines, focusing on microtia and reconstruction methodologies. This review utilized three databases: PubMed, Scopus, and Web of Science. Results: The etiology involves both genetic and environmental factors and can occur as part of a syndrome or as an isolated condition. Clinically, it has esthetic and functional implications, potentially leading to conductive hearing loss. A multidisciplinary approach is essential for treatment, which includes surgical reconstruction using autologous cartilage or synthetic prostheses. Advances in bioengineering and 3D printing offer new, less invasive solutions. Conclusions: This review aims to synthesize current knowledge on microtia, focusing on tissue engineering for auricular reconstruction, identifying research gaps, evaluating techniques, and providing a resource for clinicians to improve decision-making and foster further research.

Keywords: congenital deformity; auricular reconstruction; surgical reconstruction; autologous cartilage; synthetic prostheses; 3D printing; tissue engineering

1. Introduction

An underdeveloped or absent auricle is the result of a congenital malformation of the external ear known as microtia. It occurs with an incidence of approximately 1 in 6000 to 12,000 live births and can be unilateral (more common) or bilateral [1]. Microtia is estimated to affect around 1.46 percent of 10,000 children worldwide [2–4].

Children with this illness may suffer from psychosocial issues such as elevated anxiety, social isolation, and low self-esteem [5]. It is often associated with external auditory canal atresia, resulting in hearing problems that range from mild to severe, depending on the degree of malformation and the presence of other abnormalities in the middle and inner ear [5].

There are no definitive answers to the etiology of microtia, but it is believed to be due to a combination of genetic and environmental factors [6]. Anomalies can be isolated or associated with other syndromes, such as Goldenhar syndrome or Treacher–Collins syndrome [7]. Although studies have identified several genes that could be involved, it is challenging to establish a clear etiological framework due to the complexity of genetic and environmental interactions [8].

In clinical practice, microtia has esthetic and functional implications, with the potential for conductive hearing loss due to the absence or malformation of the auditory canal and ossicular structures [9]. Clinicians can rely on the Jahrsdoerfer grading scale as an invaluable tool in the preoperative evaluation of patients with congenital aural atresia, providing critical insights that assist in selecting the most appropriate surgical procedure [10]. The treatment of microtia requires a multidisciplinary team consisting of geneticists, otolaryngologists, audiologists, and plastic surgeons to address the functional and esthetic requirements of the patients [11]. The treatment for microtia consists of surgical interventions to reconstruct the auricle and to create or repair the auditory canal [12]. Reconstruction can be conducted with either autologous cartilage, which is typically harvested from the patient's ribs, or with synthetic prostheses [12]. The latest developments in bioengineering and 3D printing can potentially offer more personalized and less invasive solutions for treating this condition [13].

This review of the literature is intended to synthesize current knowledge on microtia, with a particular emphasis on the use of tissue engineering for auricular reconstruction. The review is intended to identify research gaps, assess the efficacy of different tissue engineering techniques, and provide a comprehensive resource for clinicians. By highlighting recent advances and comparing traditional and innovative methods, this review hopes to assist in clinical decision-making, foster cross-disciplinary cooperation, and encourage further research and development in the field.

2. Materials and Methods

A systematic approach was used to identify, analyze, and synthesize the relevant literature in accordance with PRISMA guidelines. Searches were conducted in electronic databases (such as PubMed) from 10 April to 30 November 2024. To compile the reference list, MeSH terms and free-text words were used, as reported in Appendix A, filtered by past 5 years (2019–2024). The included articles were thoroughly reviewed to identify additional relevant studies. Dr. Fracaro and Dr. Hellies independently evaluated the full texts of the articles based on the inclusion criteria after removing duplicates from all titles and abstracts. Following discussions with all authors, the reviewers reached a consensus. The inclusion criteria for the studies were as follows: (i) a description of microtia in terms of pathology and epidemiology; (ii) a description of the clinical treatment of microtia and its efficacy; and (iii) an explanation of the innovative treatments proposed, such as tissue engineering. The exclusion criteria were as follows: (i) reviews and systematic reviews; (ii) non-original studies, such as recommendations, letters, editorials, conference papers, and book chapters; and (iii) studies not written in English.

3. Results

Data Collection and Screening

A total of 151 titles were retrieved from PubMed. Records not found, records not written in English, books, and duplicates were excluded from the selection process, resulting in 107 titles. By screening the full texts of these articles, we were able to apply the inclusion/exclusion criteria, excluding 15 studies and adding 11 records (articles) as potentially relevant to the topic. Ultimately, 103 records were deemed eligible for this review. The PRISMA flow diagram in Figure 1 illustrates the progression of the information through the various stages of this literature review.

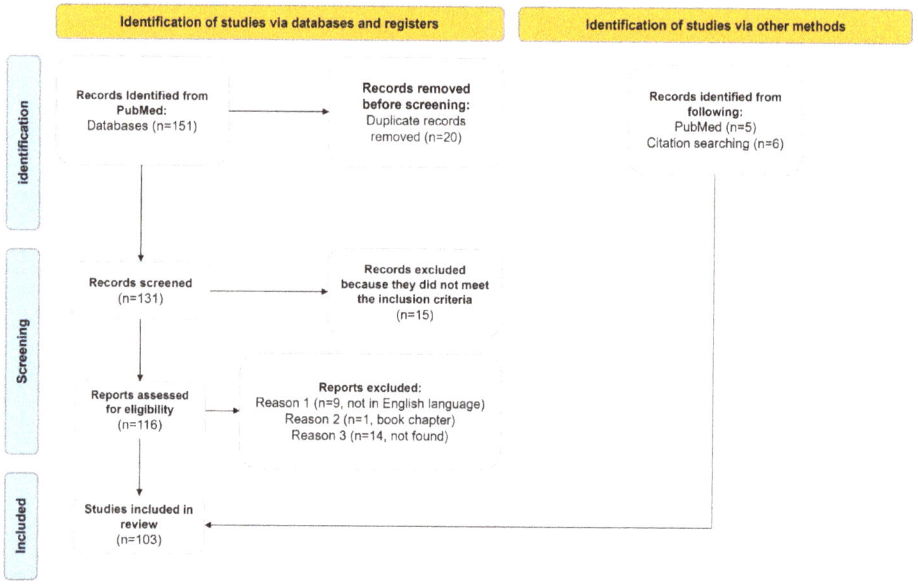

Figure 1. PRISMA 2020 flow diagram for this new systematic review which included searches of databases and other sources.

4. Discussion

4.1. General Description of Microtia

Microtia is a congenital condition characterized by the abnormal development of the external ear during the fetal stage. Its severity varies from minor deformities to the complete absence of the auricle.

This disease is classified into four grades based on severity: Grade I involves minor malformations with nearly normal anatomy, while Grade II shows partial auricular development. Grade III presents severe hypoplasia, often with a lobular remnant, and is the most common type. Grade IV (anotia) refers to the complete absence of the external ear (Figure 2). This classification guides the development of treatment strategies [5,14–16].

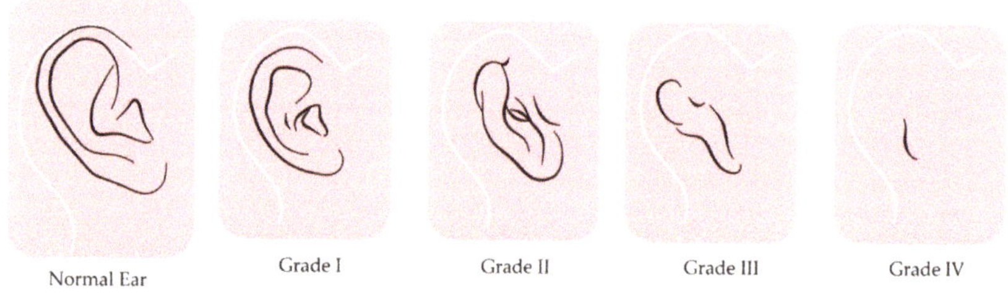

Figure 2. The image shows a normal ear alongside the four grades of microtia, ranging from mild structural changes (Grade I) to the complete absence of the external ear (Grade IV, anotia).

Microtia is more prevalent in males than females, and 90% of cases are unilateral, with a predominantly diseased right side [5].

Psychosocial effects, such as depression, anxiety, and decreased self-esteem, are commonly experienced in affected patients [17].

4.1.1. Development

Microtia is characterized by a malformation in the auricular cartilage, including folding, curling, or incomplete development, indicating that there are some abnormal steps in the cartilage development process.

Microtia auricular cartilage undergoes varying degrees of hypoplasia during early embryonic stages. It results from altered embryonic development and defective neural crest cell migration in the first and second branchial arches. The external ear begins to form around the sixth week of pregnancy, as six small nodules from the first and second arches merge. By the 12th week, the development of the auricle is completed [18].

Auricular cartilage exhibits distinct biochemical properties that influence its biomechanical behavior. For instance, the glycosaminoglycan content is higher in auricular cartilage, along with notable differences in the levels of hyaluronic acid and chondroitin sulfate. Additionally, auricular cartilage demonstrates a reduced elastin expression of elastin and an uneven collagen distribution, further distinguishing it from normal auricular cartilage [18].

4.1.2. Genetic Studies

Approximately 40% of patients with microtia exhibit additional structural abnormalities as part of the syndrome, which may involve chromosomal abnormalities or single-gene mutations [19].

There are some genes that have been identified as directly involved in microtia, such as PLCB4, GNAI3, HOXA2, DHODH, and TBX1 [20].

HOXA2 plays a critical role in the development of the second branchial arch and mutations are linked to autosomal recessive microtia, directly affecting auricle formation.

TBX1 regulates pharyngeal arch development, which is crucial for craniofacial structures. This gene is found in 22q11.2 deletion syndrome (DiGeorge syndrome), where microtia is a common feature.

Then, there are some genes involved or indirectly involved in syndromic forms such as: ROBO1/ROBO2; SIX1/SIX5, which is linked to branchio-oto-renal (BOR) syndrome where microtia is a key feature; and CHUK, involved in embryogenesis and whose mutations can lead to developmental abnormalities, including ear defects [21].

4.1.3. Epidemiological Studies

Epidemiological research has identified various factors that contribute to the development of microtia, including viral infections during early pregnancy, preeclampsia, environmental influences, and genetic predispositions.

The pathogenic mechanism of microtia is multifactorial and progresses through multiple stages. Recent genomic studies on congenital non-syndromic microtia have revealed the involvement of noncoding RNAs, such as microRNAs and long noncoding RNAs, in its development.

Increasing evidence highlights the diverse roles of ncRNAs, particularly enhancer RNAs, which are synthesized as active enhancers and influence gene expression by modulating chromatin structure and function.

Despite these findings, further research is required to validate these functions [22].

4.1.4. Treatment and Tissue Engineering

Traditional auricular reconstruction relies on autologous costal cartilage, which is considered the standard due to its biocompatibility and structural stability. However, cartilage harvesting carries risks such as pneumothorax, scarring, and reduced elasticity over time.

Innovative techniques focus on bioengineered cartilage scaffolds and 3D printing, enabling the creation of customized structures with reduced invasiveness. Additionally, the use of bioengineered skin substitutes and growth factors enhances integration and improves esthetic and functional outcomes. While promising, these approaches require further studies to ensure long-term clinical efficacy [23].

4.2. Current Surgical Techniques in Clinical Practice, Efficacy, and Limitations

Auricular reconstruction for microtia is a complex surgical challenge that requires an integrated approach, considering technical, biological, and esthetic aspects. In recent years, several studies have introduced innovative techniques to improve functionality, esthetics, and the management of postoperative complications.

In the following section, various key aspects related to current surgical techniques in auricular reconstruction and their results in terms of efficacy and limitations will be discussed.

4.2.1. Use of Autologous Cartilage

Autologous costal cartilage is considered the gold standard for auricular reconstruction in microtia due to its biological and mechanical properties, which provide a stable and long-lasting structure, ensuring a satisfactory esthetic outcome [24–27]. Its biological compatibility eliminates the risk of rejection and immunological complications, making it a reliable and widely adopted choice [28,29]. Numerous studies have confirmed its long-term efficacy, such as that of Griffin (2020), which highlights the superior mechanical properties of costal cartilage compared to other options. Griffin's study emphasizes that costal cartilage exhibits greater stiffness and robustness, making it ideal for auricular reconstruction. In fact, costal cartilage has a significantly higher Young's modulus of elasticity (11.43 MPa) compared to auricular cartilage (2 MPa) [24].

Recent studies, such as those by Yan (2019), Ladani (2018), and Park (2023), confirm that costal cartilage better conforms to the anatomical structure of the patient, enabling the creation of a rigid and resilient three-dimensional framework that replicates the complexity of the external ear [25,28,30]. Specifically, Yan (2019) and Ladani (2018) describe the well-established technique of harvesting cartilage from the sixth, seventh, and eighth ribs, selecting segments based on length, quality, and conformation, to construct a framework that faithfully reproduces auricular anatomy. These segments are chosen for their elasticity and strength, which allows the design of a robust support capable of adapting to the patient's movements and ensuring long-term durability [28,30]. Beyond dimensions, the biomechanics of costal cartilage are fundamental: it must be soft enough to be sculpted yet rigid enough to maintain its shape [26,31].

Intraoperative preparation plays a crucial role in the success of the procedure. The proper dissection and management of the donor site are essential to minimize the risk of complications [28,30]. Park (2023) analyzed the long-term outcomes of secondary auricular reconstruction in patients with unsatisfactory results from primary microtia reconstruction, identifying complications such as lump deformities (91 cases), deficient convolution (19 cases), and the absence of structures with scarred mastoid skin (22 cases) [25,32]. Secondary auricular reconstruction using autologous costal cartilage yielded favorable esthetic results and manageable complications. Outcomes, evaluated using a four-point Likert scale, showed that 42% of the patients presented excellent results, while the 36% presented only good results [25].

A further significant contribution came from Asirova's study (2023), which used CT scans to analyze the characteristics of the costal cartilage, suggesting the identification of the optimal surgical timing for reconstruction [26]. This aspect was crucial to ensure higher material quality and resistance, reducing the risk of postoperative complications and improving long-term esthetic outcomes [26]. According to this study, the optimal age for auricular reconstruction with autologous costal cartilage is from 10 years onwards, not only because the cartilage has reached an adequate size but also because the contralateral ear can be used as a model, allowing for the creation of an ear of the same size as the healthy one [26].

Autogenous cartilage also enables the detailed replication of auricular subunits through meticulous carving, reducing material requirements while achieving natural and harmonious results [33,34]. For instance, Luo et al. [29] documented successful single-stage reconstructions in 98 patients with congenital microtia, demonstrating stable and proportionate auricular morphology with minimal donor site complications. Outcomes rated as excellent or good were observed in 94 cases, with only minor issues such as hypertrophic scarring or pigmentation observed in a few patients during a 28.5-month follow-up period. Saha (2023) [35] showed a unique case of microtia associated with dextrocardia, situs inversus totalis, butterfly vertebra, and hemivertebra, describing the technical considerations necessary to optimize safety and outcomes for surgical reconstruction in such an extraordinary context. The suitability of the left or right rib cartilage for constructing the auricular frame during auricular reconstruction in pediatric patients examined by Sun (2022) [36] showed that the rib cartilage from the left side, especially the sixth rib, was generally more suitable for auricular reconstruction in pediatric patients with microtia. Anatomical abnormalities of the superficial temporal artery (STA) branches in patients with microtia and the implications for auricular reconstruction using a temporoparietal fascia (TPF) flap were described by Nguyen [37]; partial flap necrosis and facial damage were more frequent when the frontal arterial branch was within 5 mm of the facial nerve or when there was permanent nerve damage. The study of Sun (2024) [38] was a meta-analysis comparing the effectiveness of two methods of auricular reconstruction in patients with microtia: reconstruction with expanded flaps versus non-expanded flaps. The results suggested that auricular reconstruction with non-expanded flaps offers a better overall therapeutic effect, with minor postoperative complications in various key categories.

4.2.2. Operative and Postoperative Complications

The use of costochondral cartilage shows positive outcomes, with a progressive reduction in complications as the surgeon gains experience. Nevertheless, complications can arise during surgery or in the postoperative period, including esthetic concerns and patient dissatisfaction (Figure 3).

The complication rate is approximately 10%, primarily occurring during the first surgical phase, consistent with other studies, such as Torres (2021), which reported a complication rate of 16% [39]. Sharma (2024) [40] analyzed early postoperative complications in patients undergoing ear reconstruction for microtia. The results showed that alloplastic implants had a higher complication rate compared to cartilage grafts (8.6% vs. 2.8%) and an increased independent risk of wound complications.

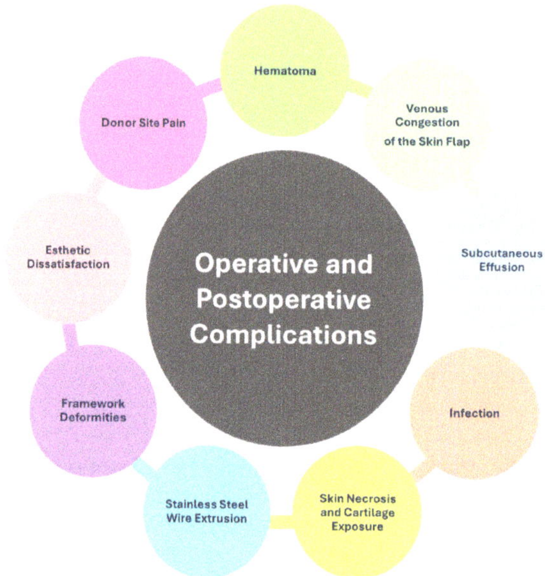

Figure 3. Summary of potential postoperative complications.

Hematoma

Hematoma is a common complication within the first postoperative day, caused by subcutaneous hemorrhage. To prevent this, meticulous intraoperative hemostasis, postoperative observation, and the use of suction drains are critical. The application of a compressive dressing for one day and, in some cases, hyperbaric oxygen therapy can facilitate the absorption of hematoma. This complication occurs in 1.4% of cases and accounts for 70% of all complications. Risk factors include imprecise hemostasis and unstable awakening from anesthesia. Proper surgical technique is essential [41].

Venous Congestion of the Skin Flap

Venous congestion manifests as a bluish discoloration occurring during the first or second postoperative day. Treatment involves small perforations with a hypodermic needle, the application of topical heparin to prevent clot formation, and hyperbaric oxygen therapy to improve circulation and recovery. This complication is attributed to the inappropriate dimensions of the subcutaneous pedicle and destruction of subcutaneous vascular networks [41].

Subcutaneous Effusion

A retrospective study concerning 1296 affected sides found 55 cases of subcutaneous effusion, including 24 cases using Nagata's method and 31 cases with the expanded single-flap method. The effusion occurred within five days after drainage tube removal. The expanded single-flap method was more prone to effusion due to the greater scope of the framework compared to that of the modified Nagata method. Patients were successfully treated with the indwelling needle puncture drainage method combined with continuous negative pressure [42].

Infection

Infections at the surgical site typically present as abnormal erythema, swelling, abscesses, and surgical wound dehiscence, usually 1 to 2 weeks after surgery. Treatment includes drainage, irrigation, intravenous antibiotics, and hyperbaric oxygen therapy. Infections account for 0.5% of complications, with a higher risk in patients with conchal-type microtia due to insufficient sterile measures and the improper use of prophylactic antibiotics [41].

Skin Necrosis and Cartilage Exposure

Skin necrosis and cartilage exposure, particularly in areas such as the helix, tragus, and incisura, occur in 22.7% of cases. For exposure areas smaller than 10 mm^2, conservative treatments are applied, while larger areas require surgical intervention with skin flaps or grafts. This complication is associated with sharp cartilage edges, excessive protrusion, or vascular destruction during dissection [41,43,44]. Notably, these cases can occur years after surgery. For instance, one study reported a spontaneous auricular abscess with exposed cartilage 20 years post-reconstruction [45].

Stainless Steel Wire Extrusion

The extrusion of stainless steel wire, which is used to secure the cartilage framework during the first stage of microtia reconstruction, is another complication. This is especially common at the helix root. To reduce extrusion, thinner wires (0.20 mm instead of 0.25 mm) are recommended, with removal during follow-up or the second surgical phase. This complication represents 17% of cases and is related to the use of thick wires or improper placement [41].

Framework Deformities

In adult patients with calcified or fragile cartilage, fractures of the eighth costal cartilage may occur during helix construction, either intraoperatively or during follow-up. Prevention involves modifying the carving technique, using the outer edge of the framework body as the helix, and reinforcing attachment points on the upper curved section. Framework deformities represent 8.8% of complications and are caused by the improper handling of hardened cartilage, delayed follow-up, or improper patient positioning [41].

Esthetic Dissatisfaction

Esthetic dissatisfaction is another possible complication, often requiring secondary revision surgery. A study of 24 cases identified the importance of tailoring revision techniques to the local soft tissue conditions of the reconstructed ear to achieve satisfactory results [41,46,47].

Donor Site Pain and Deformities

Pain at the autologous donor site is an accessory complication. An effective solution proposed in one study involved administering local analgesics to the donor area, similarly to the techniques used for rib fractures, with good results in improving recovery time and quality of life [48]. Instead, Yang et al. [49] examined the thoracic deformities that might arise following rib cartilage harvesting for auricular reconstruction in patients with microtia. To address this issue, the authors proposed a solution involving autologous dermofat transplantation to restore chest symmetry. This technique offered an effective approach to enhance both the esthetic appearance and symmetry of the chest.

Excessive Hair on Reconstructed Skin

Excess hair growth on reconstructed skin is a potential esthetic issue, especially when skin expanders are used. Studies have demonstrated that both long-pulsed 800 nm diode lasers and intense pulsed light (IPL) are safe and effective methods for hair removal during all stages of ear reconstruction. Significant results have been achieved after 2–3 sessions [50,51].

4.2.3. Innovative Surgical Techniques

In addition to traditional corrective techniques, several studies have explored innovative approaches for auricular reconstruction, including the use of cartilage molding, cadaveric material harvesting, and alloplastic materials such as resorbable plates or titanium supports.

Cartilage Molding

The application of a 3D-printed mold for the reconstruction of the auricular scaffold by using an endogenous environment was described by Wei et al. (2023) [52]. The regeneration of the constructed auricolar pavilion exploited the perichondrial flap from the sixth to eigth costal cartilage. After 6–8 months, the mold was removed, and the shaped cartilage was implanted at the final site. The results were satisfactory both esthetically and in terms of the quality of the reconstructive material. The study involved five patients, three of whom completed long-term follow-up.

Cadaveric Material

The harvesting of costal cartilage from cadavers represents a solution to the problem of material scarcity, particularly in children, while avoiding the need for double surgical intervention and associated complication at the donor site. A protocol was presented in which cadaveric costal cartilage was sterilized, sculpted, and subsequently implanted. The dense extracellular matrix (ECM) of allogeneic cartilage prevented lymphocyte migration into the transplanted tissue, inhibiting immune detection and limiting the immune response [53].

Simultaneous Reconstruction with Transcutaneous Bone Conduction Implant

Chan et al. (2019) evaluated the feasibility of simultaneous auricular reconstruction with the implantation of a bone-conduction hearing aid [54]. They showed that the approach is safe and effective and this combination might improve both esthetics and auditory function. This study presented a novel auricular prosthesis integrating a cartilage conduction hearing aid (CC-HA) using 3D data processing for patients with microtia. Preclinical evaluations showed minimal acoustic differences between the CC-HA alone and its combination with the prosthesis, with no clinical relevance. The APiCHA system offered a non-invasive, functional, and esthetic solution for hearing restoration [55].

Innovative Sculpting and Shaping Strategies

Advanced techniques have been proposed for the harvesting, sculpting, and utilization of costal cartilage in Grade I and Grade II microtia. Specifically, Gu et al. (2023) [56] described a method for the reconstruction of the helix and antihelix, which ensured the good preservation of the costal perichondrium and the use of resorbable sutures. The esthetic outcome was judged satisfactory by 100% of the 65 patients, without significant complications.

Other researchers proposed personalized modifications applied to the sculpting of different ear parts, based on the individual patients' characteristics [57]. These modifications upgraded structural stability, esthetic appearance, and the durability of the results during follow-up. Some complications had to be managed postoperatively. The described techniques offered flexibility and adaptability but required further measures to minimize postoperative risks and ensure symmetry in the final result. An alternative method was reported by Park et al. (2021) [58] using a V-Y advancement of a temporal triangular flap to obtain additional soft tissue without the use of a tissue expander. There were no specific complications after the first surgical stage, but one patient had complications after the second stage (auricular elevation). The authors reported that most of the patients reported excellent esthetic results, with satisfactory convolution. The average number of operations required to complete the reconstruction was two, lower than the conventional method using a tissue expander. Other researchers evaluated the clinical efficacy of a surgical method combining a cross-flap with autologous auricular cartilage grafting in the treatment of type I-III microtia [59]. The proposed method was effective in treating type I-III microtia, making this surgical approach feasible for correcting this deformity. In the study [60], the issue of "lop ear" was addressed, characterized by an insufficient helix and scapha, a poorly developed antihelix, and helix folding. Methods to resolve this issue were proposed based on the severity of "lop ear". More severe cases of "lop ear" were considered a type of conchal microtia. Lesta Compagnucci et al. described separating the implanted cartilaginous framework using fascial flaps and a dermal template to create an auriculocephalic sulcus. This technique reduced operative time, preserved fascia for future use, and minimized scarring with similar complication rates [61].

Plates and Titanium Supports

Li et al. (2023) proposed an innovative technique to improve ear projection and elevation in microtia reconstruction, utilizing a retroauricular fascial flap that enveloped two titanium structures [62]. These structures served as supports, aiding in achieving a stable and well-defined projection of the reconstructed ear. In this way, exclusive reliance on costal cartilage, which may not always be sufficient, was avoided. The technique, performed in a total of 51 patients with unilateral microtia (age range: 9–35 years), demonstrated satisfactory results in creating an esthetically pleasing ear with solid posterior elevation and natural projection [62].

Material Quantification

Li et al. (2024) proposed a method for quantifying the available costal cartilage in patients to optimize the surgical process and reduce the risk of material insufficiency during harvesting [63].

4.2.4. Surgical Advances for Esthetic Improvement

In recent years, surgical techniques for ear reconstruction in patients with microtia have made significant advances, aimed at improving esthetic and functional outcomes, reducing complications, and optimizing long-term stability. The most notable innovation was the introduction of the posterior auricular artery perforator (PAAP) free flap, described by Banda (2020), which enhanced the vascularization of the reconstructed tissues, reducing the risk of necrosis and improving the stability of the auricular implant [64]. This technique was particularly effective in the reconstruction of the retroauricular sulcus, a critical area for achieving functional and esthetically pleasing results [64].

Simultaneously, innovations in cartilage framework sculpting techniques have led to significant esthetic improvements. Luo et al. (2023), in a study concerning 98 patients, introduced modifications to the sculpting of costal cartilage, optimizing the definition of the helix and antihelix, as well as the angulation and symmetry of the auricular pavilion [29]. These improvements allowed for reconstructions more faithful to the natural anatomy of the ear, positively affecting both the esthetic appearance and functionality of the pavilion [29]. Similarly, Mazeed et al. (2020) proposed the use of a complete ring-shaped cartilage framework with accentuated curves, which improved structural stability and definition of the tragus and concha, preventing postoperative deformities and optimizing esthetic results [65].

The use of costal cartilage continues to be a fundamental resource in ear reconstruction. Wang et al. (2021) introduced a crescent-shaped cartilage graft to improve the retroauricular contour [66], or a three-stage technique involving the creation of a cartilage framework and the use of a skin flap, demonstrating satisfactory esthetic and functional results despite the inherent challenges in adult ear reconstruction [67].

An innovation of Firmin's technique improved earring insertion in patients undergoing ear reconstruction [68]. This modification allowed for the creation of a specific area for the earring hole without compromising esthetics, thereby improving patient satisfaction and postoperative quality of life [68].

Other innovative approaches include the study by Lee et al. (2023), which integrated a superficial temporal fascial flap with a costal cartilage graft, improving the vascularization and stability of the auricular framework [69]; a three-stage approach showed superior results in the study by Xu et al. (2019), who developed advanced three-dimensional modeling of the cartilage framework, leading to significant improvements in esthetic results and a reduction in complications [70]. Furthermore, studies conducted by Ibrahiem (2023) optimized conchal-type microtia reconstruction and the elevation of the ear [71] with improvements in esthetics and functionality and a reduction in scarring [72,73]. Greene et al. [74] proposed an alternative approach for ear elevation, where an advanced x-y flap improved the integrity and contour of the reconstructed auricular sulcus and a modification to the Nagata technique improved the projection and esthetics of reconstructed ears [75]. This study involved 38 patients (39 ears), whose ages ranged from 6 to 34 years, with an average follow-up of approximately 33.6 months. A proportion of 15.4% of the results were rated as excellent and 41% as good. A total of 79.9% of patients or their families reported being satisfied. No cases of flap necrosis or hypertrophic scars were observed. Low complication rates were found: a mismatch in skin color (7.7%), unacceptable thickness (5.1%), and the presence of hair or stretch marks (10.3%). Other researchers focused on auricular reconstruction, particularly optimizing rib cartilage carving techniques to create esthetically harmonious auricular structures. In 406 patients, 112 ears were rated as "excellent". A design based on these data allowed for the creation of a harmonious and well-defined three-dimensional ear, with minimal risk of complications [76].

4.2.5. Tissue Expansion

In recent years, the combination of tissue expansion and advanced reconstructive techniques has significantly improved the management of microtia by optimizing the use of available tissues and reducing the need for skin grafts. These techniques have also improved the esthetic and functional outcomes of auricular reconstruction.

An innovative approach developed by Wang et al. (2021) combined tissue expansion with autologous auricular reconstruction. The technique, applied to 104 patients (average age of 12 years), involved two stages: the use of an expander to stretch the mastoid skin, followed by a Y-shaped incision to separate the earlobe from other skin structures. In the second stage, a cartilage framework was inserted into the expanded area, optimizing the projection and definition of the cranio-auricular sulcus. This approach reduced complications and improved patient satisfaction [77].

A similar technique developed by Chen et al. (2020) employed an extended postauricular flap combined with tissue expansion, eliminating the need for skin grafts and reducing visible scarring. Applied to 106 patients, this technique achieved a success rate of 93.4%, improving vascularization and reducing complications compared to traditional methods [78].

Liang et al. (2023) optimized the design and positioning of tissue expanders, improving skin coverage and esthetic outcomes, as this technique reduced skin necrosis and enhanced tissue integration, resulting in a high degree of patient satisfaction [79].

The tissue expansion technique for auricular reconstruction has several limitations, including a prolonged treatment period, high saline volume requirements, and restricted patient selection based on skin elasticity and thickness. Reduced vascularization of the expanded flap increases the risk of necrosis and ischemia, while excessive tissue expansion may promote hair growth in the reconstructed area. Additionally, insufficient cartilage rigidity can compromise the definition of the auriculocephalic sulcus. The risk of infections, the need for corrective procedures, and the multiple surgical stages make this technique complex and less widely applicable [77–79].

4.3. Tissue Engineering in Otology Application

A tissue engineering approach to auricular reconstructions could offer the potential to overcome the limitations of both autologous and alloplastic transplants.

Tissue engineering has facilitated the creation of cartilaginous frameworks tailored to individual patient needs. However, several challenges persist, including the requirement for large quantities of chondrogenic cells, addressing the complexities of resistance to deformation forces, and ensuring long-term framework stability [1]. It is important to note that auricular cartilage is predominantly composed of collagen and elastin fibers embedded in a proteoglycan gel, imparting viscoelastic properties to the structure [1]. For this reason, the graft must not only meet structural demands concerning the shape substitute, including its dimensions and thickness, but also replicate the mechanical properties of the auricle, which has been demonstrated to have different stiffnesses across different regions [24].

Thus, to closely mimic native tissue, an ideal scaffold should possess several key characteristics, such as an adequate pore size, a large surface area, a degradation rate balanced with the rate of tissue regeneration, sufficient mechanical strength to maintain its predesigned shape, biocompatibility, and positive interactions with cells. These include promoting cellular adhesion, migration, proliferation, and differentiation to achieve optimal integration between the biomaterial and tissue (Figure 4).

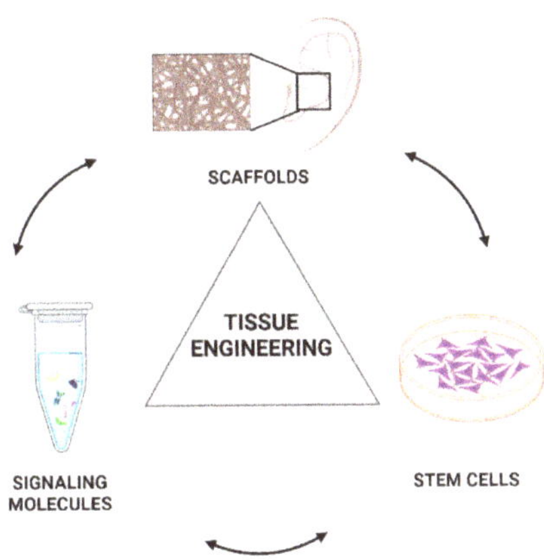

Figure 4. The tissue engineering triad: scaffolds, cells, and signaling molecules are the three key elements of tissue engineering. Scaffolds act as the structural framework for tissue formation, cells play a role in tissue regeneration, and signaling molecules regulate cellular activities and interactions. Created in BioRender. https://BioRender.com/i36c115, accessed on 28 February 2025.

For this reason, one of the most promising approaches involves directly fabricating the 3D shape [80] of the ear using the scaffold material, potentially incorporating cells within the construct. While these strategies show promise, they are not without limitations. However, the major challenge in engineered cartilage for auricular reconstruction is the exceptionally high number of chondrocytes required. Cartilage from microtia patients does not provide a sufficient number of functional chondrocytes to meet this demand. Furthermore, even when chondrocytes are cultured in monolayers, achieving the necessary amount remains problematic due to the progressive loss of their chondrogenic potential during the in vitro expansion [1].

Regarding 3D reconstruction, a current procedure involves the reuse of microtic tissues. Specifically, vestigial cartilage can successfully replace costal cartilage to enhance the projection and three-dimensional contour of the reconstructed ear, yielding satisfactory results in terms of shape, symmetry, and stability, with high patient satisfaction [81]. Additionally, Jacob et al. found that microtic perichondrocytes exhibit similar chondrogenic properties to chondrocytes in vitro, suggesting their potential as a promising cell source for auricular reconstruction [6]. However, results are contradictory; while some studies report robust cartilage formation by microtic chondrocytes, others demonstrate their inferior chondrogenic capacity and the formation of disorganized structures in 3D cell culture models [17].

In the following sections, synthetic, hybrid/composite, and biological materials utilized for external ear reconstruction will be described, along with their respective advantages and limitations. Additionally, scaffold-free techniques, which represent an alternative approach in tissue-engineered auricular reconstruction, will also be discussed (Figure 5).

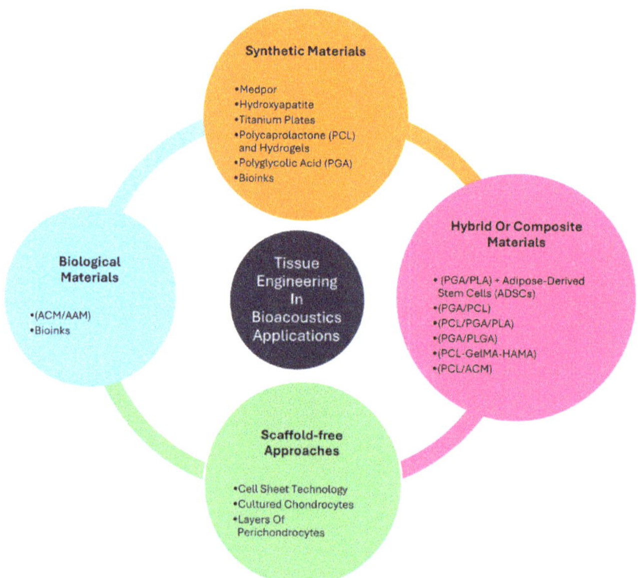
Synthetic Materials
•Medpor
•Hydroxyapatite
•Titanium Plates
•Polycaprolactone (PCL) and Hydrogels
•Polyglycolic Acid (PGA)
•Bioinks
Biological Materials
•(ACM/AAM)
•Bioinks
Tissue Engineering In Bioacoustics Applications
Hybrid Or Composite Materials
• (PGA/PLA) + Adipose-Derived Stem Cells (ADSCs)
•(PGA/PCL)
•(PCL/PGA/PLA)
•(PGA/PLGA)
•(PCL-GelMA-HAMA)
•(PCL/ACM)
Scaffold-free Approaches
•Cell Sheet Technology
•Cultured Chondrocytes
•Layers Of Perichondrocytes

Figure 5. Overview of materials used in bioacoustics, including synthetic biomaterials, hybrid and composite materials, and scaffold-free approach for tissue engineering applications.

4.3.1. Synthetic Materials

Synthetic materials have emerged as alternatives to autologous rib cartilage for auricular reconstruction, addressing the issue of donor site morbidity associated with cartilage harvesting. Among these, porous high-density polyethylene (pHDPE), commercially known as Medpor (Stryker, Kalamazoo, MI, USA), is one of the most extensively utilized materials. Its interconnected pore structure (average pore size ~150 μm) promotes fibrovascular ingrowth, facilitating integration with surrounding tissues. Compared to autologous cartilage, pHDPE offers advantages such as reduced operative time, the possibility of use in younger patients, and the elimination of complications related to rib cartilage harvesting [82]. A 3D mirror-image prefabricated template served as a three-dimensional reference for surgeons to meticulously sculpt the MEDPOR framework. This step ensured that the final implant closely matched the intricate details and spatial relationships of the patient's normal ear, enhancing both precision and symmetry in the reconstruction process [83]. However, compared to autologous cartilage, Medpor exhibits lower biocompatibility, as it lacks the ability to integrate dynamically with the surrounding biological environment. Unlike native tissue, it does not undergo remodeling or adapt to physiological changes over time. Additionally, Medpor does not grow with the patient, which may limit its suitability for pediatric applications, where long-term tissue adaptation is crucial for optimal functional and esthetic outcomes.

Wei et al. (2023) [84] proposed a novel method for repairing cartilaginous defects by using hyaluronic acid (HA) and leveraging the self-regenerative potential of the intercostal rib space. HA was used to 3D print auricular models, which were then implanted in the chest wall to promote tissue repopulation. An incision was made between the sixth and eighth ribs, and the perichondrium was detached from the costal cartilage. The costal cartilage from the 6th to 8th ribs was removed, and the perichondria were sutured together to form a connected perichondral flap. The HA ear-shaped mold was then sutured to this flap. After 6–8 months, the HA molds were removed. The histological examination of the explanted tissue revealed ear-shaped, cartilage-like structures, with H&E staining showing the presence of chondrocytes. Alcian blue staining indicated a rich matrix of glycosaminoglycans (GAGs). Immunohistochemistry with anti-collagen type II antibodies demonstrated that GAG-positive regions also contained collagen type II. The study reported no significant adverse events from implanting the HA mold into the chest cavity, and no adverse reactions were observed even when the auricular implant was used as a replacement for a damaged ear [84].

An important factor when selecting a support material is its suitability for pediatric patients, who constitute a substantial proportion of recipients. Unlike HA or titanium plates, resorbable plates do not require removal, which represents a critical advantage.

While the mechanical strength of resorbable plates is lower compared to HA or titanium, this limitation is less consequential in auricular reconstruction due to the minimal physical stress exerted on the plates [84].

Resorbable plates are recognized for their favorable attributes, offering robust and long-lasting support without excessive volume. They provide reliable fixation with a reduced risk of dislocation when secured with screws. To avoid the drawbacks of previous synthetic materials, biodegradable scaffolds, such as those combining polymers like polycaprolactone (PCL) with hydrogels, were explored to promote tissue regeneration while providing temporary mechanical support. These materials degraded over time as new cartilage formed, avoiding the long-term presence of foreign materials [85].

In detail, the PCL was used for ear reconstruction by using a 3D printing technique mimicking the real cartilage, where pores of 2 mm were incorporated to enable the placement of diced cartilage, which facilitated its regeneration. The same technique was applied in a clinical trial with five patients with unilateral microtia who underwent a two-stage ear reconstruction [85]. The 3D-printed cartilage, designed to be non-identical to the other ear graft, demonstrated to provide appropriate vascularity and a reduced infection risk [85].

Another biodegradable material is polyglycolic acid (PGA), which has a fibrous structure with a large surface area and significant pore volume, facilitating tissue integration and cell regeneration, particularly chondrocyte growth. The degradation byproduct, glycolic acid, is non-toxic and is metabolized through the tricarboxylic acid cycle, ultimately being excreted as water and carbon dioxide, with a portion also eliminated in the urine. For this reason, PGA was selected as the suitable scaffold for chondrocyte culture, subcutaneous implantation, and cartilage development, aiming to optimize the number of passages and environmental conditions to promote the growth of auricular cartilage from a folded PGA scaffold while preserving its biofunctional properties [86]. In the study, the optimization of autologous chondrocyte seeded PGA scaffolds was investigated for ear cartilage regeneration starting from a small ear biopsy. In particular, PGA scaffolds seeded with chondrocyte + mesenchymal stem cells (MSCs) subcutaneously implanted in immunosuppressed mice did not grow after two months of implantation, but when the same material seeded with chondrocytes was implanted in rabbits, cartilage 10 times larger than the original PGA scaffold formed, with biofunctional and mechanical properties similar to ear cartilage. For ear reconstruction, an innovative approach based on 3D printing was recently proposed, enabling the creation of patient-specific auricular structures to closely mimic the unique anatomy of the individual. Imaging techniques such as CT or MRI scans of the healthy contralateral ear can generate highly personalized 3D models for reconstruction purposes. These methods allow for the more precise replication of natural ear morphology, enhancing esthetic and functional outcomes. One of the primary challenges in 3D bioprinting for auricular reconstruction lies in balancing the scaffold's structural integrity with its ability to support cell migration and tissue integration. Materials like bioinks composed, for example, of hydrogels are commonly used due to their biocompatibility and capacity to encapsulate cells like chondrocytes that are responsible for cartilage production [85].

The framework for 3D-printed ears has been demonstrated to offer several advantages compared to autologous costal cartilage or synthetic alternatives like porous polyethylene. First, it allows for the precise, patient-specific modeling of the ear, facilitated by CT scans that generate highly accurate designs. This method enables the detailed extraction of unaffected ear structures by differentiating surrounding tissues and isolating specific auricular cartilage regions [85]. Second, there is no risk of complications related to donor sites. Third, the choice of implant materials can be tailored to achieve the desired balance between mechanical strength and biodegradability. Additionally, the approach ensures the preservation of the subcutaneous pedicle, enhances the vascularity of the skin flap, and lowers the likelihood of postoperative issues such as infections, skin necrosis, or implant exposure. Lastly, PCL-based 3D printing for auricular the reconstruction of the cartilage delivers robust mechanical properties with gradual biodegradability, making it a highly effective solution [86].

Poly-ε-caprolactone was used by Velasquillo et al. (2024) [87] as well. In detail, 3D-printed Poly-ε-caprolactone scaffolds coated with a fibrin hydrogel and seeded with human microtia chondrocytes were subcutaneously implanted into the dorsal region of 10 athymic mice. As a control group, five mice received scaffolds coated only with fibrin hydrogel, without chondrocytes. Four weeks after implantation, the authors reported no signs of extrusion or skin necrosis, and the ear-like structures remained stable at the implantation site [87].

Specifically, in the seeded group, white cartilage-like tissue was formed, exhibiting sufficient mechanical strength to retain its initial shape despite the pressure exerted by the overlying skin. Additionally, the grafts in this group were covered with a thin layer of vascularized tissue that resembled native tissue. Conversely, in the unseeded group, no new tissue formation was observed, and the fibrin hydrogel had resorbed. However, the grafts showed no signs of degradation but were notably more rigid compared to those of the seeded group [87].

4.3.2. Hybrid or Composite Materials

Hybrid materials represent a specific subset within composite materials. Composites, by definition, are created by combining two or more distinct materials that differ in their chemical and/or physical properties, resulting in a new material with enhanced characteristics tailored for a specific application. A widely accepted description of hybrid materials highlights the synergistic integration of organic and inorganic components at the microscopic (molecular) level, leading to the development of unique material properties. The close integration of inorganic, organic, or a combination of both types of components enables the formation of advanced materials with improved functionalities compared to the properties of their individual constituents [88].

In auricle reconstruction, polyglycolic acid/polylactic acid (PGA/PLA) composite scaffolds have gained significant attention in tissue-engineered ear reconstruction due to their versatility and ease of molding. For example, in a canine model, PGA demonstrated promising results in terms of cell adhesion compared to other biodegradable polymers, promoting cartilage regeneration. However, it did not exhibit entirely satisfactory mechanical properties, as it failed to maintain the complex three-dimensional shape of a normal ear. For this reason, the combination of PGA with PCL was investigated to merge the positive attributes of both materials [89], creating a hybrid scaffold as stated elsewhere [88]. Specifically, a PCL scaffold with suitable rigidity and ear-like geometry was coated with PGA nanofibers. Nanofibers were chosen over conventional PGA because it was shown that PGA, during hydrolysis, increased environmental acidity, leading to inflammation and localized tissue destruction impeding regeneration. In contrast, the PGA/PCL material treated with ethanol improved hydrophilicity and thus cell adhesion to the scaffold. Thus, PGA/PCL might have facilitated cartilage regeneration, while untreated scaffolds led to a progressive loss of chondrocytes and proteoglycans [89].

Wu et al. (2024) [90] further advanced this technique by repopulating PGA/PLA scaffolds with adipose-derived stem cells (ADSCs), which are readily accessible, abundant, and possess strong chondrogenic potential. These ADSCs, co-cultured with chondrocytes overexpressing RhoA, demonstrated enhanced extracellular matrix (ECM) deposition and improved chondrocyte organization. The overexpression of RhoA in microtia chondrocytes significantly promoted cell migration, facilitating more uniform tissue formation. Coculturing mesenchymal stem cells and chondrocytes has consistently been shown to be a superior strategy compared to using individual cell types, as it leverages the synergistic effects of both cell populations in cartilage tissue engineering. In their study, Wu et al. implanted PGA/PLA constructs populated with modified ADSCs and MSCs subcutaneously in nude mice. After four weeks of preculture in vitro, the scaffolds exhibited the significant degradation of PGA/PLA fibers, leaving behind well-organized tubular structures and cartilage-like tissue. Histological analysis revealed a highly organized chondrocyte arrangement in constructs utilizing RhoA-overexpressed cells, further demonstrating the potential of this approach for auricular cartilage regeneration.

Resorbable plates were then used in a two-stage microtia reconstruction for 12 patients to provide structural support during auricular elevation [91]. The plates were gradually resorbed, eliminating the need for rigid materials such as metals or autologous cartilage. This approach resulted in a well-defined contour and appropriate elevation of the ear, with promising long-term outcomes, including a low complication rate and high patient satisfaction. In another study, Mukherjee et al. (2021) [8] aimed to improve the biocompatibility of PLA by developing scaffolds composed of polycaprolactone (PCL), gelatin methacrylate (GelMA), and hyaluronic acid methacrylate (HAMA) to address the limitations of traditional PCL-based materials. These scaffolds were enzymatically treated with lipase to enhance porosity, promote accelerated in vivo degradation, and improve biocompatibility compared to that of untreated PCL, used as a control. The materials were evaluated in vivo by subdermal implantation in sheep, representing a non-functional test. While there was no skin irritation, the formation of a pseudocapsule and limited tissue integration were observed, alongside a modest inflammatory response characterized by multinucleated giant cells surrounding the scaffolds. Importantly, the PCL-GelMA-HAMA scaffolds demonstrated greater cell repopulation compared to pure PCL. Despite this improvement, both materials elicited an inflammatory response, highlighting the need for further optimization to reduce adverse reactions while maintaining biocompatibility and promoting effective tissue integration [8].

Moreover, hybrid materials have recently gained attention as a promising approach to address both mechanical and biological challenges using the 3D printing approach. This technique combines the precision and strength of a stiffer polymer for structural support with biologically derived materials that create a favorable microenvironment for cell proliferation and differentiation, including stem cells. By co-printing these components, hybrid printing ensures both mechanical integrity and the biological functionality necessary for effective tissue regeneration. Despite these successes, the presence of heterogeneous cartilage regions and residual fibrous tissue highlights the need for further optimization of scaffold preparation techniques and a comprehensive evaluation of their biosafety. These findings underscore the importance of fine-tuning bioink formulations and enhancing printing methodologies to achieve uniform cartilage regeneration and minimize adverse tissue responses [88].

4.3.3. Biological Materials

Auricular cartilage consists of an extracellular matrix (ECM) rich in type II collagen, proteoglycans, elastin, and water, providing structural strength and elasticity. Type II collagen forms the primary structural framework, while elastin fibers, arranged in a fine network interspersed with collagen fibrils, contribute to the deformability essential for auricular function. Mimicking this composition is a key objective in the development of biological substitutes for auricular cartilage reconstruction. By replicating these properties, it is possible to create a replacement that closely resembles native cartilage, providing an effective solution for restoring cartilage in conditions such as microtia.

To study the state of cartilage, various techniques can be employed, as demonstrated in the study of elastic and hyaline cartilage derived from laryngeal cartilage. In Gentilin et al. (2023), a protocol for whole-organ decellularization was developed to preserve the integrity of the ECM [92]. The efficiency of decellularization and the preservation of ECM components were evaluated using a range of staining and microscopy techniques. Hematoxylin/eosin (H&E), Masson Trichrome, and DAPI staining, along with DNA quantification, were utilized to assess decellularization efficiency. For collagen detection and quantitative assessment, Van Gieson staining, Picrosirius Red staining (PRS) and multiphoton laser scanning microscopy (MPM) were employed. Additionally, polarized PRS was used to investigate the collagen network, while Weigert staining and MPM were applied for elastin detection and quantification. This comprehensive approach ensured a thorough evaluation of the decellularization process and the preservation of critical ECM components [92].

Collagen, the most prevalent component of the ECM, has emerged as a promising biomaterial for scaffolds in cartilage reconstruction, particularly in cases such as auricular repair for microtia. Its advantages include low immunogenicity, a porous structure conducive to cell infiltration, and excellent biocompatibility. However, collagen-based scaffolds often lack the mechanical stiffness required for the structural demands of auricular cartilage. Additionally, biologically derived tissues, such as the decellularized cartilage matrix (ACM) and allograft adipose matrix (AAM), represent some of the most advanced materials under investigation for auricular tissue engineering. In recent years, decellularized tissues have garnered significant interest due to their promising applications in various fields of tissue reconstruction. The decellularization process involves the removal of cellular components from xenogeneic tissues, which are readily available in large quantities. This approach renders the material non-immunogenic while preserving the extracellular matrix structure, making it suitable for recellularization with the patient's own cells. Such properties make decellularized tissues particularly attractive for the development of scaffolds that combine biocompatibility, mechanical stability, and the potential for functional integration [93–98].

In detail, for the reconstruction of ears affected by microtia, decellularized adipose tissue was tested in the form of disks measuring 15 mm in diameter and 2 to 3 mm in thickness as a scaffold for the co-seeding of porcine auricular chondrocytes and stem cells derived from cadavers' adipose tissue (two ratios were evaluated, specifically 1:5 and 1:9) [99–102]. Compared to the two control groups (i.e., each cell type seeded individually on the scaffold), which remained viable even 10 weeks post-seeding, the co-seeding of chondrocytes and adipose tissue-derived stem cells facilitated the deposition of the ECM, particularly collagen type II. Among the tested ratios, the 1:9 ratio (chondrocytes–adipose tissue-derived stem cells) yielded the most favorable results [96].

4.3.4. Scaffold-Free Approach

Scaffold-free techniques have been introduced for cartilage engineering, including cell sheet technology, aggregate culture methods, and self-assembly processes. Aggregate culturing involves cultivating cells in a way that facilitates cell-to-cell interactions, resulting in the formation of free-floating cell clusters in a two-dimensional configuration. Cell sheet technology, instead, employs cultured monolayers that are manipulated thermally or physically, sometimes with or without enzymatic cleavage, depending on the mandrel used. This method enables the stacking of multiple layers resulting in a thicker tissue construct. In contrast, the self-assembly process enables chondrocytes to aggregate naturally without external energy input. This approach leverages intrinsic free energy and cellular tension to promote adhesion between cells, simulating the mesenchymal condensation observed during natural cartilage development [94,96,99]. It should be noted that the scaffold-free approach generates a cartilage block that requires surgical sculpting to achieve the desired shape, rather than a preformed three-dimensional auricular structure. This method produces cartilage without the use of external supporting materials; however, the resulting tissue necessitates additional shaping to attain the final anatomical configuration.

Cultured chondrocytes obtained from autologous cartilage represent a potential alternative to the traditional use of rib cartilage in auricular reconstruction. Protocols have been developed for extracting chondrocytes from small tissue samples, expanding them in vitro, and generating cartilage constructs suitable for implantation. Despite these advancements, studies using immunosuppressed mice to test chondrocyte-laden scaffolds or hydrogels (e.g., PGA, polylactic acid, or their blends) have not successfully produced the cartilage volume required to recreate a full-sized human ear. This shortfall is partly attributed to the limited regenerative capacity of chondrocytes from microtia tissue compared to those from healthy cartilage. To overcome these challenges, it is essential to refine cell expansion methods, optimize passage numbers, and establish ideal culture conditions for the effective use of microtia-derived autologous chondrocytes in tissue-engineered scaffolds [99].

Enomura et al. (2020) [103] proposed the use of three layers of perichondrocytes harvested from microtia patients to create a scaffold-free construct capable of regenerating elastic cartilage when implanted in NOD/SCID mice. Although promising, this approach resulted in the formation of cartilage measuring only 1 cm^3, whereas a cartilage volume of 10 cm^3 is required to effectively treat microtia [100].

5. Conclusions

Microtia reconstruction remains a challenging yet evolving field that bridges traditional surgical techniques with groundbreaking advancements in tissue engineering and regenerative medicine. While autologous costal cartilage grafting has long been regarded as the gold standard due to its biocompatibility and structural stability, its limitations—such as donor-site morbidity, technical complexity, and variability in outcomes—highlight the critical need for innovative alternatives.

Recent advancements in tissue engineering, including 3D bioprinting, scaffold-based constructs, and stem cell therapies, are transforming the landscape of auricular reconstruction. These technologies offer precise, personalized solutions that reduce invasiveness, improve esthetic outcomes, and minimize complications. For instance, bioengineered scaffolds and decellularized matrices provide platforms for cartilage regeneration, while 3D-printed models enable preoperative planning and mirror-image reconstructions that enhance symmetry and patient satisfaction. Additionally, the integration of endogenous stem cells and growth factors holds immense potential for promoting tissue regeneration and long-term stability.

Despite these promising developments, significant challenges remain. The standardization of protocols, optimization of biomaterials, and validation of long-term clinical outcomes are essential to ensure the safety and efficacy of these emerging techniques. Furthermore, broader accessibility to advanced technologies, particularly in regions with high microtia incidence, must be addressed to maximize their global impact.

In summary, this review underscores the transformative potential of tissue engineering in microtia reconstruction, emphasizing its role in overcoming the limitations of traditional methods. By advancing regenerative approaches and integrating cutting-edge technologies, we can pave the way for more effective, less invasive, and highly personalized treatments, ultimately improving quality of life for patients with microtia.

Author Contributions: Conceptualization, L.A. and G.A.; methodology, S.F. and F.H.; investigation, S.F., F.H., A.T., M.T. and M.C.; data curation, S.F. and F.H.; writing—original draft preparation, L.A., G.A., S.F., F.H., A.T., M.T. and M.C.; writing—review and editing, L.A., G.A., S.F., F.H., A.T., M.T, M.C., G.M., A.B. and E.Z.; visualization: L.A., G.A., S.F., F.H., A.T., M.T., G.M., A.B. and E.Z.; supervision, L.A. and G.A.; funding acquisition: L.A. All authors have read and agreed to the published version of the manuscript.

Funding: This research was funded by University of Padua, grant number 2024DNS1DOR-00973.

Acknowledgments: Figures were created under license using BioRender.com. https://biorender.com/, accessed on 28 February and 18 March 2025.

Conflicts of Interest: The authors declare no conflicts of interest.

Appendix A

Specific search details were entered into the query boxes of each database as follows.

Pub med

(((ear cartilage) AND (congenital microtia)) OR (("Congenital Microtia"[Mesh]) AND ("Ear Cartilage"[Mesh]))) OR ((("Congenital Microtia"[Mesh]) AND ("Tissue Engineering"[Mesh])) OR ((congenital microtia) AND (tissue engineering))) AND ((y_5[Filter]) AND (english[Filter])) AND ((y_5[Filter]) AND (english[Filter]))

Scopus

(TITLE-ABS-KEY (congenital AND microtia) AND TITLE-ABS-KEY (ear AND cartilage)) OR (TITLE-ABS-KEY (congenital AND microtia) AND TITLE-ABS-KEY (tissue AND engineering)) AND PUBYEAR > 2018 AND PUBYEAR < 2025 AND (LIMIT-TO (DOCTYPE, "ar")) AND (LIMIT-TO (LANGUAGE, "English"))

Web of Science

Congenital microtia (All Fields) and ear cartilage (All Fields) or congenital microtia (All Fields) and tissue engineering (Author) and 2020 or 2021 or 2022 or 2023 or 2024 or 2019 (Publication Years) and Article (Document Types) and English (Languages)

References

1. Khan, N.; Zaki, D.P.; Brown, W.E.; Halaseh, F.F.; Willette, D.; Ziegler, M.; Athanasiou, K.A.; Widgerow, A.D. Tissue Engineering Auricular Cartilage: A Review of Auricular Cartilage Characteristics and Current Techniques for Auricular Reconstruction. *J. Craniofacial Surg.* **2024**, *35*, 768–778. [CrossRef] [PubMed]
2. Mastroiacovo, P.; Corchia, C.; Botto, L.D.; Lanni, R.; Zampino, G.; Fusco, D. Epidemiology and Genetics of Microtia-Anotia: A Registry Based Study on over One Million Births. *J. Med. Genet.* **1995**, *32*, 453–457. [CrossRef]
3. Huang, Y.; Zhao, H.; Wang, Y.; Bi, S.; Zhou, K.; Li, H.; Zhou, C.; Wang, Y.; Wu, W.; Peng, B.; et al. The Application and Progress of Tissue Engineering and Biomaterial Scaffolds for Total Auricular Reconstruction in Microtia. *Front. Bioeng. Biotechnol.* **2023**, *11*, 1089031. [CrossRef] [PubMed]
4. Zielinska, D.; Fisch, P.; Moehrlen, U.; Finkielsztein, S.; Linder, T.; Zenobi-Wong, M.; Biedermann, T.; Klar, A.S. Combining Bioengineered Human Skin with Bioprinted Cartilage for Ear Reconstruction. *Sci. Adv.* **2023**, *9*, eadh1890. [CrossRef]
5. Truong, M.T.; Liu, Y.-C.C.; Kohn, J.; Chinnadurai, S.; Zopf, D.A.; Tribble, M.; Tanner, P.B.; Sie, K.; Chang, K.W. Integrated Microtia and Aural Atresia Management. *Front. Surg.* **2022**, *9*, 944223. [CrossRef] [PubMed]
6. Jakob, Y.; Kern, J.; Gvaramia, D.; Fisch, P.; Magritz, R.; Reutter, S.; Rotter, N. Suitability of Ex Vivo-Expanded Microtic Perichondrocytes for Auricular Reconstruction. *Cells* **2024**, *13*, 141. [CrossRef]
7. Gardner, O.F.W.; Agabalyan, N.; Weil, B.; Ali, M.H.I.; Lowdell, M.W.; Bulstrode, N.W.; Ferretti, P. Human Platelet Lysate Enhances Proliferation but Not Chondrogenic Differentiation of Pediatric Mesenchymal Progenitors. *Cytotherapy* **2023**, *25*, 286–297. [CrossRef]
8. Mukherjee, P.; Chung, J.; Cheng, K.; Gupta, R.; Haag, H.; Williams, Z.; Wallace, G. Invitro and Invivo Study of PCL-Hydrogel Scaffold to Advance Bioprinting Translation in Microtia Reconstruction. *J. Craniofacial Surg.* **2021**, *32*, 1931–1936. [CrossRef]
9. Chen, X.; Zhang, R.; Zhang, Q.; Xu, Z.; Xu, F.; Li, D.; Li, Y. Microtia Patients: Auricular Chondrocyte ECM Is Promoted by CGF through IGF-1 Activation of the IGF-1R/PI3K/AKT Pathway. *J. Cell Physiol.* **2019**, *234*, 21817–21824. [CrossRef]
10. Shonka, D.C.; Livingston, W.J.; Kesser, B.W. The Jahrsdoerfer Grading Scale in Surgery to Repair Congenital Aural Atresia. *Arch. Otolaryngol. Head. Neck Surg.* **2008**, *134*, 873–877. [CrossRef]
11. Wu, Y.; Liu, W.; Li, J.; Shi, H.; Ma, S.; Wang, D.; Pan, B.; Xiao, R.; Jiang, H.; Liu, X. Decreased Tiam1-mediated Rac1 Activation Is Responsible for Impaired Directional Persistence of Chondrocyte Migration in Microtia. *J. Cell Mol. Med.* **2024**, *28*, e18443. [CrossRef] [PubMed]
12. Otto, I.A.; Simone, A.; Malda, J.; Kon, M.; Breugem, C.C. Engaging Stakeholders in Bioprinting Research: Views and Concerns of Microtia Patients' Parents on Bioprinted Auricular Cartilage. *J. Plast. Reconstr. Aesthetic Surg.* **2020**, *73*, 2239–2260. [CrossRef] [PubMed]
13. Chen, J.; Huang, T.; Liu, R.; Wang, C.; Jiang, H.; Sun, H. Congenital Microtia Patients: The Genetically Engineered Exosomes Released from Porous Gelatin Methacryloyl Hydrogel for Downstream Small RNA Profiling, Functional Modulation of Microtia Chondrocytes and Tissue-Engineered Ear Cartilage Regeneration. *J. Nanobiotechnol.* **2022**, *20*, 164. [CrossRef]
14. Padilla-Cabello, J.; Moral-Munoz, J.A.; Santisteban-Espejo, A.; Velez-Estevez, A.; Cobo, M.J.; Martin-Piedra, M.A. Analysis of Cognitive Framework and Biomedical Translation of Tissue Engineering in Otolaryngology. *Sci. Rep.* **2023**, *13*, 13492. [CrossRef]
15. McDaniel, S.L.; Hollatz, A.J.; Branstad, A.M.; Gaskill, M.M.; Fox, C.A.; Harrison, M.M. Tissue-Specific DNA Replication Defects in Drosophila Melanogaster Caused by a Meier-Gorlin Syndrome Mutation in Orc4. *Genetics* **2020**, *214*, 355–367. [CrossRef]
16. Guo, F.; Lin, L.; Yu, X.; Song, Y.; Yang, Q.; He, L.; Pan, B.; Jiang, H. Classification of the Concha-Type Microtia and Their New Suitable Treatment Strategies without Autogenous Costal Cartilage Grafting. *Int. J. Pediatr. Otorhinolaryngol.* **2020**, *130*, 109801. [CrossRef]
17. Lam, D.D.; Hegde, N.V.; Patel, D.D.; Lakeland, D.L.; Guardino, N.; Kochhar, A.; Mariani, F.V. Histological Assessment of Microtia Cartilage, a Potential Source of Autograft Tissue in Ear Reconstruction. *J. Anat.* **2024**, *245*, 339–345. [CrossRef] [PubMed]
18. Yang, J.; He, L. Mass Spectrometric Characterization of Metabolites in Ear Cartilage. *Ann. Plast. Surg.* **2020**, *85*, 76–82. [CrossRef]
19. Liu, W.; Wu, Y.; Ma, R.; Zhu, X.; Wang, R.; He, L.; Shu, M. Multi-Omics Analysis of a Case of Congenital Microtia Reveals Aldob and Oxidative Stress Associated with Microtia Etiology. *Orphanet J. Rare Dis.* **2024**, *19*, 218. [CrossRef]
20. Dong, W.; Jiang, H.; He, L.; Pan, B.; Lin, L.; Song, Y.; Yang, Q. Protein Profile of Ear Auricle Cartilage and the Important Role of ITGB1/PTK2 in Microtia. *Int. J. Pediatr. Otorhinolaryngol.* **2020**, *137*, 110235. [CrossRef]
21. Yang, R.; Chu, H.; Yue, H.; Mishina, Y.; Zhang, Z.; Liu, H.; Li, B. BMP Signaling Maintains Auricular Chondrocyte Identity and Prevents Microtia Development by Inhibiting Protein Kinase A. *eLife* **2024**, *12*, RP91883. [CrossRef] [PubMed]

22. Liu, Y.; Zhao, Y.; Lin, L.; Yang, Q.; Zhang, L. Differential Expression of Noncoding RNAs Revealed Enhancer RNA AC016735.2 as a Potential Pathogenic Marker of Congenital Microtia Patients. *J. Craniofacial Surg.* **2024**, *35*, 787–793. [CrossRef]
23. Zielinska, D.; Yosef, H.K.; Zollitsch, T.; Kern, J.; Jakob, Y.; Gvaramia, D.; Rotter, N.; Pontiggia, L.; Moehrlen, U.; Biedermann, T.; et al. Characterization of Distinct Chondrogenic Cell Populations of Patients Suffering from Microtia Using Single-Cell Micro-Raman Spectroscopy. *Biomedicines* **2023**, *11*, 2588. [CrossRef] [PubMed]
24. Griffin, M.F.; O'Toole, G.; Sabbagh, W.; Szarko, M.; Butler, P.E. Comparison of the Compressive Mechanical Properties of Auricular and Costal Cartilage from Patients with Microtia. *J. Biomech.* **2020**, *103*, 109688. [CrossRef]
25. Park, C. Total Rebuilding of the Ear after Unsatisfactory Initial Microtia Reconstruction: 30-Year Experience Using Autogenous Costal Cartilage Framework. *J. Plast. Reconstr. Aesthetic Surg.* **2023**, *86*, 174–182. [CrossRef]
26. Asirova, G.; Wynands, J.; Frolov, S.; Almeida, D.; Davydenko, P.; Madina, S. Optimal Surgical Timing for Ear Reconstruction with Autologous Cartilage: Analysis of the Computed Tomography Scan Characteristics of the Ribs. *J. Plast. Reconstr. Aesthet. Surg.* **2024**, *88*, 15–23. [CrossRef]
27. Kim, A.; Moon, J.; Lim, S.Y.; Oh, K.S. The Interchondral Joints of Thorax in Microtia Surgery: Classification and Fabrication Strategies. *Ann. Plast. Surg.* **2021**, *87*, 98–104. [CrossRef]
28. Ladani, P.S.; Valand, R.; Sailer, H. Ear Reconstruction Using Autologus Costal Cartilage: A Steep Learning Curve. *J. Maxillofac. Oral. Surg.* **2019**, *18*, 371–377. [CrossRef]
29. Luo, K.; Chen, Z.; Jiang, Z.; Cai, S.; Zhou, Y.; Cui, W.; Sheng, Y.; Lin, Y.; Chen, Y.; Cai, Z. Ear Reconstruction Stage I: Minor Modifications in Sculpting the Auricle Support Using the 7th and 8th Costal Cartilages. *J. Plast. Reconstr. Aesthet. Surg.* **2023**, *84*, 357–364. [CrossRef]
30. Yan, H.; Zhang, G.; Liu, W.; Wang, N.; Liu, Z. Different Methods of Fabricating Cartilaginous Ear Framework in Children With Microtia According to the Length of the Eighth Costal Cartilage Intraoperatively. *J. Craniofacial Surg.* **2019**, *30*, 1425–1429. [CrossRef]
31. Xing, W.; Qian, J.; Wang, B.; Wang, Y.; Hu, J.; Zhang, Q. Auricular Reconstruction with Modified Expanded Two-Flap Method in Goldenhar Syndrome: 7-Year Experiences. *Int. J. Pediatr. Otorhinolaryngol.* **2020**, *139*, 110228. [CrossRef]
32. Mao, X.; Li, X.; Jia, J.; Kang, D.; Miao, Y.; Lu, Z.; Hu, Z. Validity and Reliability of Three-dimensional Costal Cartilage Imaging for Donor-site Assessment and Clinical Application in Microtia Reconstruction Patients: A Prospective Study of 22 Cases. *Clin. Otolaryngol.* **2020**, *45*, 204–210. [CrossRef] [PubMed]
33. Li, D.; Zhang, R.; Zhang, Q.; Xu, Z.; Xu, F.; Li, Y.; Sun, N.; Wang, C. A Novel Method of Naturally Contouring the Reconstructed Ear. *Plast. Reconstr. Surg.* **2014**, *133*, 1168–1174. [CrossRef]
34. Yang, J.; Lin, L.; Zhang, Y.; Wang, Y.; Cui, L.; He, L. The Regenerated Tissue at the Donor Site After Costal Cartilage Harvest for Auricular Reconstruction. *J. Craniofacial Surg.* **2019**, *30*, e490–e494. [CrossRef]
35. Saha, S.; Singh, A.; Mohammad, A.; Chauhan, S.; Chinta, K.; Singhal, M. Don't Play It by Ear: Technical Considerations to Optimize Outcome and Procedural Safety of Congenital Microtia Reconstruction in a Dextrocardia Patient With Situs Inversus Totalis, Butterfly Vertebra, and Hemivertebra. *Eplasty* **2023**, *23*, e57.
36. Sun, H.; Huang, Q.; Dong, W.; Yang, Q. Differences between Bilateral Costal Cartilage in Patients with Microtia: A Retrospective Study Using Three-Dimensional Imaging. *Plast. Reconstr. Surg.* **2022**, *149*, 939–942. [CrossRef] [PubMed]
37. Nguyen, H.H.; Vu, D.D.; Ngo, L.M.; Tran, H.T.T. Anatomical Variant of the Superficial Temporal Artery in Temporoparietal Fascia Flap for Microtia Reconstruction. *J. Plast. Reconstr. Aesthet. Surg.* **2024**, *91*, 105–110. [CrossRef]
38. Sun, P.; Wang, C.; Luan, F.; Pan, B. Comparison of Auricle Reconstruction with Expanded Flaps and Auricle Reconstruction with Non-Expanded Flaps in Patients with Microtia: A Meta-Analysis. *Ear Nose Throat J.* **2024**, *103*, NP351–NP359. [CrossRef] [PubMed]
39. Torres, I.; Martinez, J.D.C.; Sanabria, R.; González, L.V.; Díaz-Báez, D. Postoperative Safety and Satisfaction in Patients With Microtia. *J. Oral. Maxillofac. Surg.* **2021**, *79*, 472.e1–472.e9. [CrossRef]
40. Sharma, R.K.; DeSisto, N.G.; Ortiz, A.S.; Landeen, K.C.; Yang, S.F.; Stephan, S.J.; Patel, P.N. Early Postoperative Complications in Microtia Reconstruction: An Analysis of the NSQIP-P Database. *Laryngoscope* **2024**, *134*, 1214–1219. [CrossRef]
41. Xu, Z.; Li, T.; Zhang, R.; Zhang, Q.; Xu, F.; Li, D.; Li, Y.; Chen, X. Strategies for the Treatment of Auricular Complications after the First Stage of Autologous Cartilage Microtia Reconstruction. *Plast. Reconstr. Surg.* **2022**, *150*, 157e–167e. [CrossRef] [PubMed]
42. Guo, R.; Liu, T.; Wang, B.; Zhang, Q. Management Strategy of Local Subcutaneous Effusion After Auricle Reconstruction. *Ear Nose Throat J.* **2023**, *102*, 667–672. [CrossRef] [PubMed]
43. Sasaki, K.; Sasaki, M.; Oshima, J.; Nishijima, A.; Aihara, Y.; Sekido, M. Salvaging Exposed Microtia Cartilage Framework with Negative Pressure Wound Therapy. *J. Plast. Reconstr. Aesthetic Surg.* **2021**, *74*, 1355–1401. [CrossRef] [PubMed]
44. Fujioka, M.; Fukui, K.; Yoshino, K.; Noguchi, M.; Murakami, R. Salvage of Ear Framework Exposure Following Autologous Microtia Reconstruction: Repair Strategy for Each Location of Exposure. *Cleft Palate Craniofacial J.* **2023**, *60*, 1172–1175. [CrossRef]
45. Tuang, G.J.; Mansor, M.; Abdullah, A. An Unusual Delayed Complication of Rib Graft Microtia Reconstruction After Two Decades: A Case Report. *Indian. J. Otolaryngol. Head. Neck Surg.* **2022**, *74*, 3671–3674. [CrossRef]

46. Yue, X.; Jiang, H.; Pan, B.; He, L.; Dong, W.; Yang, Q. Secondary Surgery for the Unsatisfactory Auricle after Auricular Reconstruction. *Int. J. Pediatr. Otorhinolaryngol.* **2022**, *154*, 111043. [CrossRef]
47. Reinisch, J.F.; van Hövell Tot Westerflier, C.V.A.; Gould, D.J.; Tahiri, Y.T. Secondary Salvage of the Unsatisfactory Microtia Reconstruction. *Plast. Reconstr. Surg.* **2020**, *145*, 1252–1261. [CrossRef]
48. Xiang, G.; Chen, C.; Chen, K.; Liu, Q.; Sun, X.; Huang, Y.; Huang, L.; Jin, J.; Shang, J.; Yang, D. Comparing the Analgesic Effects Between the Pre- and Post-Costal Cartilage Harvest Cohorts Using Ultrasound-Guided Deep Serratus Anterior Plane Block in Children with Microtia Undergoing Auricular Reconstruction: A Randomized Clinical Trial. *Aesthetic Plast. Surg.* **2024**, *48*, 1846–1854. [CrossRef]
49. Yang, Y.; Yue, X.; Yu, X.; Pan, B. Free Dermofat Grafting for Chest Deformity in Microtia Reconstruction. *J. Plast. Reconstr. Aesthet. Surg.* **2023**, *82*, 130–136. [CrossRef]
50. Liu, Y.; Huang, L.; Feng, Y.; Huo, M.; Lin, L.; Zhang, L. Utilization of Intense Pulsed Light for Hair Removal in Pediatric Auricular Reconstruction Using Tissue Expander: A Retrospective Cohort Study. *Medicine* **2023**, *102*, e33736. [CrossRef]
51. Yang, Q.; Qiang, S.; Fan, X.; Guo, S.Z.; Yin, Y.; Li, T.; Dang, H.; Dong, L.W.; Song, B.Q. Clinical Application of Long-Pulsed 800-Nm Diode Laser Depilation Technology on Microtia Reconstruction in 965 Patients. *Aesthetic Plast. Surg.* **2024**, *48*, 2155–2161. [CrossRef]
52. Wei, J.; Baptista-Hon, D.T.; Wang, Z.; Li, G.; Herrler, T.; Dai, C.; Liu, K.; Yu, B.; Chen, X.; Yang, M.; et al. Bioengineered Human Tissue Regeneration and Repair Using Endogenous Stem Cells. *Cell Rep. Med.* **2023**, *4*, 101156. [CrossRef]
53. Palacios, J.F.; Hazkour, N.; Robinson, E.; Swami, P.; Smith, L.; Grande, D.; Bastidas, N. Primary Ear Reconstruction Using Cadaveric Costal Cartilage. *Ann. Plast. Surg.* **2023**, *90*, S547–S551. [CrossRef] [PubMed]
54. Chan, K.-C.; Wallace, C.G.; Wai-Yee Ho, V.; Wu, C.-M.; Chen, H.-Y.; Chen, Z.-C. Simultaneous Auricular Reconstruction and Transcutaneous Bone Conduction Device Implantation in Patients with Microtia. *J. Formos. Med. Assoc.* **2019**, *118*, 1202–1210. [CrossRef]
55. Nishiyama, T.; Hayashi, S.; Oishi, N. A Novel Auricular Prosthesis Which Incorporates a Cartilage Conduction Hearing Aid Based on 3D Data Processing Technique: A Preclinical Evaluation. *Eur. Arch. Otorhinolaryngol.* **2022**, *279*, 3741–3744. [CrossRef] [PubMed]
56. Gu, L.; Sun, P.; Pan, B.; Jiang, H. Subtractive Thinking: A Novel Combined Application of Antihelix Reconstruction and Outer Helix Reconstruction to Treat Mild Cases of Type I to II Conchal Microtia. *J. Plast. Reconstr. Aesthet. Surg.* **2023**, *84*, 462–468. [CrossRef] [PubMed]
57. Li, Y.; Li, D.; Xu, Z.; Zhang, R.; Zhang, Q.; Xu, F.; Chen, X. New Strategies for Base Frame Fabrication in Microtia Reconstruction. *Sci. Rep.* **2021**, *11*, 15947. [CrossRef]
58. Park, H.Y.; Lee, K.-T.; Kim, E.-J.; Oh, K.S. Reconstruction of Congenital Microtia after Ear Canaloplasty Using V-Y Advancement of a Temporal Triangular Flap. *Arch. Plast. Surg.* **2021**, *48*, 614–621. [CrossRef]
59. Sun, P.; Lu, M.; Wang, C.; Pan, B.; Jiang, H. Clinical Observations of a Surgical Method Comprising a Combination of Cross Flap and Autologous Auricular Cartilage Transplantation in the Treatment of Type I to III Congenital Concha-Type Microtia. *Ear Nose Throat J.* **2024**, *103*, NP60–NP66. [CrossRef]
60. Lese, I.; Aldabbas, M.; Mazeed, A.S.; Bulstrode, N.W. Lop Ear to Conchal Microtia. *Ann. Plast. Surg.* **2022**, *88*, 188–194. [CrossRef]
61. Lesta-Compagnucci, L.; Arámburo-García, R.; Galaso-Trujillo, J.R.; Apellaniz-Campo, A.G.; Pérez-Caro, E. Morbidity in Patients With Separation of Cartilaginous Framework: Temporoparietal Fascia Flap and Treatment With Dermal Regeneration Template. *J. Craniofacial Surg.* **2020**, *31*, 107–109. [CrossRef]
62. Li, D.; Sun, J.; Zhang, R.; Xu, Z.; Zhang, Q.; Xu, F.; Li, Y.; Chen, X. Firm Elevation of the Auricle in Reconstruction of Microtia with a Retroauricular Fascial Flap Wrapping Two Titanium Plate Struts. *J. Plast. Reconstr. Aesthet. Surg.* **2023**, *83*, 134–140. [CrossRef]
63. Li, C.-L.; Xie, Y.-Z.; He, A.; Liu, N.-H.; Cui, C.-X.; Chen, Y.; Fu, Y.; Zhang, T. Quantitative Framework Fabrication with Autogenous Costal Cartilage in Microtia Reconstruction. *Laryngoscope* **2024**, *134*, 148–153. [CrossRef] [PubMed]
64. Banda, C.H.; Narushima, M.; Mitsui, K.; Danno, K.; Fujita, M.; Furuya, M.; Karakawa, R.; Ogishima, S.; Ishiura, R. Posterior Auricular Artery Free Flap Reconstruction of the Retroauricular Sulcus in Microtia Repair. *J. Plast. Reconstr. Aesthet. Surg.* **2021**, *74*, 2349–2357. [CrossRef]
65. Mazeed, A.S.; O'Hara, J.; Bulstrode, N.W. Modification of the Cartilaginous Framework for Autologous Ear Reconstruction: Construction of a Stable Complete Ring Framework with Grander Highs and Lows. *J. Plast. Reconstr. Aesthet. Surg.* **2021**, *74*, 1832–1839. [CrossRef] [PubMed]
66. Wang, Q.; Wang, Y.; Wang, M.; Li, Q.; Zhang, Q.; Zhou, X. A Modified Crescent Cartilage Block for Improving the Retroauricular Contour of the Reconstructed Ear: A Retrospective Cohort Study. *J. Plast. Reconstr. Aesthet. Surg.* **2021**, *74*, 1324–1330. [CrossRef]
67. Ma, T.; Li, L.; Wang, X.; Zhang, Z. Auricular Reconstruction in Adult Patients With Unprepared Congenital Microtia: A Single Institution's Experience. *Ann. Plast. Surg.* **2022**, *89*, 395–399. [CrossRef]
68. Parri, F.; Alonso, V.; Albert, A.; Bejarano, M.; Vicario, F.; Rubio-Palau, J. Auricular Reconstructive Surgery Improvement to the Firmin Technique for Placing an Earring. *Cleft Palate Craniofacial J.* **2019**, *56*, 1260–1262. [CrossRef]

69. Lee, J.S.; Kim, J.S.; Lee, J.W.; Choi, K.Y.; Yang, J.D.; Chung, H.Y.; Cho, B.C. Correction of Microtia with Constriction Features Using a Superficial Temporal Fascial Flap Combined with a Rib Cartilage Graft. *Arch. Plast. Surg.* **2020**, *47*, 317–323. [CrossRef]
70. Xu, Z.; Zhang, R.; Zhang, Q.; Xu, F.; Li, D.; Li, Y. New Strategies for Tragus and Antitragus Complex Fabrication in Lobule-Type Microtia Reconstruction. *Plast. Reconstr. Surg.* **2019**, *144*, 913–921. [CrossRef]
71. Xu, Z.; Li, Y.; Li, D.; Zhang, R.; Zhang, Q.; Xu, F.; Chen, X. Strategies for Ear Elevation and the Treatment of Relevant Complications in Autologous Cartilage Microtia Reconstruction. *Sci. Rep.* **2022**, *12*, 13536. [CrossRef] [PubMed]
72. Ibrahiem, S.M.S. Concha-Type Microtia: New Surgical Incision. *Aesthet. Surg. J.* **2023**, *43*, NP815–NP822. [CrossRef]
73. Li, G.; Zhang, B.; Ding, W.; Ouyang, H.; Long, X.; Fu, A.; Liu, X. Reconstruction of Concha-Type Microtia Using a Delayed Postauricular Skin Flap. *Plast. Reconstr. Surg.* **2024**, *153*, 407e–410e. [CrossRef]
74. Greene, A.K.; Sudduth, C.L. Elevation of Costal Cartilage Ear Construct for Microtia Using a V-Y Scalp Flap. *J. Craniofacial Surg.* **2020**, *31*, 1467–1468. [CrossRef] [PubMed]
75. Quang, L.X.; Linh, T.N.T.; Ha, V.T.H.; Quyen, L.V.V.; Ngoc, T.L.H.; Dung, N.T.; Nga, N.T.T.; Chen, Y.-C.; Hung, S.-H.; Dang, L.H. A Two-Flap Combination for Auricular Elevation in Microtia Reconstruction. *Plast. Reconstr. Surg.* **2023**, *151*, 991e–1001e. [CrossRef]
76. Li, D.; Zhang, R.; Xu, Z.; Zhang, Q.; Xu, F.; Li, Y.; Chen, X.; Hou, R. Ear Reconstruction: Empirical Data of 406 Cases of Carving the Convex Structures of the Framework. *Laryngoscope* **2023**, *133*, 569–575. [CrossRef]
77. Wang, B.; Guo, R.; Li, Q.; Ou, Y.; Hu, J.; Wang, Y.; Zhang, Q.; Liu, T. A Novel Two-Stage Strategy Combing Tissue Expansion and Nagata's Technique for Total Auricular Reconstruction. *J. Plast. Reconstr. Aesthet. Surg.* **2021**, *74*, 2358–2363. [CrossRef] [PubMed]
78. Chen, Q.; Zhang, J.; Wang, B.; Wang, Y.; Kang, C.; Zhang, Q. Total Auricular Reconstruction Using a Single Extended Postauricular Flap Without Skin Grafting in Two Stages: Experiences of 106 Cases. *Aesthetic Plast. Surg.* **2020**, *44*, 365–372. [CrossRef]
79. Liang, J.; Cao, T.; Wang, Y.; Wang, B.; Qian, J.; Chen, Q.; Zhang, Q. A Modified Tissue Expander Method for Ear Reconstruction in Patients with Excessively Insufficient Postauricular Skin. *Ear Nose Throat J.* **2023**, *102*, NP449–NP456. [CrossRef]
80. Landau, S.; Szklanny, A.A.; Machour, M.; Kaplan, B.; Shandalov, Y.; Redenski, I.; Beckerman, M.; Harari-Steinberg, O.; Zavin, J.; Karni-Katovitch, O.; et al. Human-Engineered Auricular Reconstruction (HEAR) by 3D-Printed Molding with Human-Derived Auricular and Costal Chondrocytes and Adipose-Derived Mesenchymal Stem Cells. *Biofabrication* **2021**, *14*, 015010. [CrossRef]
81. Badawy, M.S.; Elshahat, A. Retroposition of the Vestigial Cartilage in Patients With Microtia: A Novel Technique to Enhance Projection of the Reconstructed Ear. *J. Craniofacial Surg.* **2022**, *33*, 1197–1200. [CrossRef]
82. Guo, R.; Ying, J.; Yuan, X.; Xi, T.; Xiong, J.; Jiang, H. Novel Method for High-Density Porous Polyethylene Ear Reconstruction Stent Remodeling to Achieve High Satisfactory Outcomes. *J. Cosmet. Dermatol.* **2022**, *21*, 3486–3493. [CrossRef] [PubMed]
83. Chen, H.-Y.; Ng, L.-S.; Chang, C.-S.; Lu, T.-C.; Chen, N.-H.; Chen, Z.-C. Pursuing Mirror Image Reconstruction in Unilateral Microtia: Customizing Auricular Framework by Application of Three-Dimensional Imaging and Three-Dimensional Printing. *Plast. Reconstr. Surg.* **2017**, *139*, 1433–1443. [CrossRef] [PubMed]
84. Wei, Y.; Li, L.; Xie, C.; Wei, Y.; Huang, C.; Wang, Y.; Zhou, J.; Jia, C.; Junlin, L. Current Status of Auricular Reconstruction Strategy Development. *J. Craniofacial Surg.* **2024**, *35*, 984–992. [CrossRef]
85. Joo, O.Y.; Kim, T.H.; Kim, Y.S.; Roh, T.S.; Lee, E.-J.; Shim, J.-H.; Cho, H.W.; Yun, I.S. Fabrication of 3D-Printed Implant for Two-Stage Ear Reconstruction Surgery and Its Clinical Application. *Yonsei Med. J.* **2023**, *64*, 291–296. [CrossRef] [PubMed]
86. Melgar-Lesmes, P.; Bosch, O.; Zubajlo, R.; Molins, G.; Comfort, S.; Luque-Saavedra, A.; López-Moya, M.; García-Polite, F.; Parri Ferrandis, F.J.; Rogers, C.; et al. Optimization of 3D Autologous Chondrocyte-Seeded Polyglycolic Acid Scaffolds to Mimic Human Ear Cartilage. *Biomater. Sci.* **2023**, *11*, 3695–3708. [CrossRef]
87. Velasquillo, C.; Melgarejo-Ramírez, Y.; García-López, J.; Gutiérrez-Gómez, C.; Lecona, H.; González-Torres, M.; Sánchez-Betancourt, J.I.; Ibarra, C.; Lee, S.J.; Yoo, J.J. Remaining Microtia Tissue as a Source for 3D Bioprinted Elastic Cartilage Tissue Constructs, Potential Use for Surgical Microtia Reconstruction. *Cell Tissue Bank.* **2024**, *25*, 571–582. [CrossRef]
88. Casarin, M.; Todesco, M.; Fontanella, C.G.; Morlacco, A.; Dal Moro, F.; Bagno, A. Hybrid Materials for Tissue Repair and Replacement: Another Frontier in Biomaterial Exploitation Focusing on Cardiovascular and Urological Fields. *Processes* **2023**, *11*, 2013. [CrossRef]
89. Hirano, N.; Kusuhara, H.; Sueyoshi, Y.; Teramura, T.; Murthy, A.; Asamura, S.; Isogai, N.; Jacquet, R.D.; Landis, W.J. Ethanol Treatment of NanoPGA/PCL Composite Scaffolds Enhances Human Chondrocyte Development in the Cellular Microenvironment of Tissue-Engineered Auricle Constructs. *PLoS ONE* **2021**, *16*, e0253149. [CrossRef]
90. Wu, Y.; Wang, J.; Li, X.; Wang, K.; Huang, Z.; Wang, Q.; Fu, X.; Jiang, H.; Pan, B.; Xiao, R. Co-Culture of RhoA-Overexpressed Microtia Chondrocytes and Adipose-Derived Stem Cells in the Construction of Tissue-Engineered Ear-Shaped Cartilage. *Stem Cells* **2024**, *42*, 554–566. [CrossRef]
91. Moon, J.; Lee, J.; Oh, K.S.; Lim, S.Y. Usefulness of Resorbable Plate in Auricular Elevation in Two-Stage Microtia Reconstruction. *Int. J. Pediatr. Otorhinolaryngol.* **2023**, *171*, 111646. [CrossRef]
92. Gentilin, E.; Simoni, E.; Albertin, G.; Candito, M.R.; Sandrin, D.; Romanato, F.; Martini, A.; Nicolai, P.; Astolfi, L. Characterization of a Decellularized Rat Larynx: Comparison between Microscopy Techniques. *Ann. Anat.—Anat. Anz.* **2023**, *245*, 152020. [CrossRef]

93. Todesco, M.; Imran, S.J.; Fortunato, T.M.; Sandrin, D.; Borile, G.; Romanato, F.; Casarin, M.; Giuggioli, G.; Conte, F.; Marchesan, M.; et al. A New Detergent for the Effective Decellularization of Bovine and Porcine Pericardia. *Biomimetics* **2022**, *7*, 104. [CrossRef]
94. Casarin, M.; Fortunato, T.M.; Imran, S.J.; Todesco, M.; Sandrin, D.; Marchesan, M.; Gerosa, G.; Romanato, F.; Bagno, A.; Dal Moro, F.; et al. Preliminary In Vitro Assessment of Decellularized Porcine Descending Aorta for Clinical Purposes. *J. Funct. Biomater.* **2023**, *14*, 141. [CrossRef] [PubMed]
95. Casarin, M.; Fortunato, T.M.; Imran, S.; Todesco, M.; Sandrin, D.; Borile, G.; Toniolo, I.; Marchesan, M.; Gerosa, G.; Bagno, A.; et al. Porcine Small Intestinal Submucosa (SIS) as a Suitable Scaffold for the Creation of a Tissue-Engineered Urinary Conduit: Decellularization, Biomechanical and Biocompatibility Characterization Using New Approaches. *Int. J. Mol. Sci.* **2022**, *23*, 2826. [CrossRef]
96. Childs, R.D.; Nakao, H.; Isogai, N.; Murthy, A.; Landis, W.J. An Analytical Study of Neocartilage from Microtia and Otoplasty Surgical Remnants: A Possible Application for BMP7 in Microtia Development and Regeneration. *PLoS ONE* **2020**, *15*, e0234650. [CrossRef]
97. Yue, H.; Pathak, J.L.; Zou, R.; Qin, L.; Liao, T.; Hu, Y.; Kuang, W.; Zhou, L. Fabrication of Chondrocytes/Chondrocyte-Microtissues Laden Fibrin Gel Auricular Scaffold for Microtia Reconstruction. *J. Biomater. Appl.* **2021**, *35*, 838–848. [CrossRef]
98. Donnelly, H.; Kurjan, A.; Yong, L.Y.; Xiao, Y.; Lemgruber, L.; West, C.; Salmeron-Sanchez, M.; Dalby, M.J. Fibronectin Matrix Assembly and TGFβ1 Presentation for Chondrogenesis of Patient Derived Pericytes for Microtia Repair. *Biomater. Adv.* **2023**, *148*, 213370. [CrossRef]
99. Ziegler, M.E.; Sorensen, A.M.; Banyard, D.A.; Evans, G.R.D.; Widgerow, A.D. Improving In Vitro Cartilage Generation by Co-Culturing Adipose-Derived Stem Cells and Chondrocytes on an Allograft Adipose Matrix Framework. *Plast. Reconstr. Surg.* **2021**, *147*, 87–99. [CrossRef]
100. Uto, S.; Hikita, A.; Sakamoto, T.; Mori, D.; Yano, F.; Ohba, S.; Saito, T.; Takato, T.; Hoshi, K. Ear Cartilage Reconstruction Combining Induced Pluripotent Stem Cell-Derived Cartilage and Three-Dimensional Shape-Memory Scaffold. *Tissue Eng. Part A* **2021**, *27*, 604–617. [CrossRef]
101. Zucchelli, E.; Birchall, M.; Bulstrode, N.W.; Ferretti, P. Modeling Normal and Pathological Ear Cartilage in Vitro Using Somatic Stem Cells in Three-Dimensional Culture. *Front. Cell Dev. Biol.* **2020**, *8*, 666. [CrossRef]
102. Sakahara, D.; Yanaga, H.; Noto, M.; Fujimoto, T.; Imai, K. Long-Term Clinical Results of Two-Stage Total Ear Reconstruction of Microtia Using Autologous Cell-Engineered Chondrocytes. *Plast. Reconstr. Surg.* **2023**, *151*, 282e–287e. [CrossRef] [PubMed]
103. Enomura, M.; Murata, S.; Terado, Y.; Tanaka, M.; Kobayashi, S.; Oba, T.; Kagimoto, S.; Yabuki, Y.; Morita, K.; Uemura, T.; et al. Development of a Method for Scaffold-Free Elastic Cartilage Creation. *Int. J. Mol. Sci.* **2020**, *21*, 8496. [CrossRef] [PubMed]

MDPI AG
Grosspeteranlage 5
4052 Basel
Switzerland
Tel.: +41 61 683 77 34

Children Editorial Office
E-mail: children@mdpi.com
www.mdpi.com/journal/children

www.ingramcontent.com/pod-product-compliance
Lightning Source LLC
Chambersburg PA
CBHW062040220926
51850CB00010B/2611
* 9 7 8 3 7 2 5 8 7 3 4 2 5 *